RECOVERING FROM HEART DISEASE

HEART

RECOVERING FROM HEART DISEASE IN BODY & MIND

MEDICAL AND PSYCHOLOGICAL STRATEGIES FOR LIVING WITH CORONARY ARTERY DISEASE

BRIAN BAKER, M.B.Ch.B

PAUL DORIAN, M.D., M.Sc.

Foreword by Bretta Maloff, M.Ed., R.D.

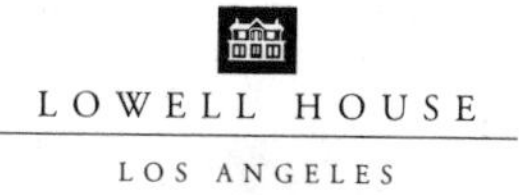

NTC/Contemporary Publishing Group

Published by Lowell House
A division of NTC/Contemporary Publishing Group, Inc.
4255 West Touhy Avenue, Lincolnwood, Illinois 60646-1975 U.S.A.

This edition published by arrangement with Random House Canada, a division of Random House Canada Limited.

Library of Congress Cataloging-in-Publication Data is available.

Printed in the United States of America

International Standard Book Number: 0-7373-0360-3

00 01 02 03 04 DHD 18 17 16 15 14 13 12 11 10 9 8 7 6 5 4 3 2 1

To Sabrina, Lisa and Natalie,
Sally, Katie, David, Lindsay and Jenny

Contents

A Note to the Reader xi
Acknowledgments xiii
Foreword xv

CHAPTER 1

Preparing for the Journey: About This Book and How to Use It

Why did we write this book? 1
Who is our intended reader? 3
How is this book different from other books on heart disease? 4

PART ONE: THE GUIDE

CHAPTER 2

Guide to the Journey: An Introduction

What you need to know about "The Guide" 11
Forum (Tony): Does awareness help? 16

CHAPTER 3

Event

What's wrong with Anna? 21
What happened? 22
What, in fact, happened to my heart? 24
What happened to me?! 27
What to expect 31
Forum (Anna): Dealing with the event 32

CHAPTER 4
Aftermath
Rose is lost 38
Where am I? 39
Where am I medically? 40
Where am I emotionally? 43
Family concerns 45
Forum (Rose): Lost and found 47

CHAPTER 5
Recuperation
Is Mary healing? 52
The body heals 54
The mind reacts 63
Family matters 72
Achieving a balance 73
Forum (Mary): Finding the path of healing 78

CHAPTER 6
Rehabilitation
What can Joe do? 85
An approach to rehabilitation 88
The fork in the road 91
The importance of adaptive denial 92
The magic of empowerment 93
The secret of empowerment: Structured activity 94
Can I prevent my CAD from recurring or progressing? 97
Family concerns 98
A guide to the rehab programs 100
Slippage 112
Forum (Joe): Getting into gear 113

CHAPTER 7

Recovery

Has Kevin recovered? 121

Home at last 123

Can I recover from CAD? 123

What is *realistic* recovery? 125

What do I still need to do? 127

The challenge of maintenance 129

Family note 130

Keeping a balance 131

Forum (Kevin): Looking back and looking forward 134

PART TWO: DIRECTIONS

CHAPTER 8

What You Need to Know about "Directions": An Introduction 145

CHAPTER 9

Heart: Key Physical Issues for Those with Heart Disease

What is heart disease? 149

What to do in an emergency 158

What happens when you go to the hospital? 160

Tests often performed on patients with heart disease 162

Surgical procedures often performed on patients with heart disease 167

Medications often prescribed for patients with heart disease 169

Your team of professionals 181

Medical research 184

Risk factors for coronary heart disease 188
Women and heart disease 203

CHAPTER 10
Mind: Key Emotional Issues for Those with Heart Disease
Anxiety 206
Depression 210
Stress and CAD 216
Stress management and the seven vulnerabilities 219
Stress and heart disease: A patient's personal view 237
When to seek counseling, and from whom 242
Psychiatric emergency 245

CHAPTER 11
Heart to Mind: Three Dialogues between Cardiology and Psychiatry about the Journey to Recovery
The third way 246
Themes of healing 252
Ready for rehabilitation 260

CHAPTER 12
Six Journeys
Tony: "What—me worry?" 265
Anna: "Repeated episodes" 270
Rose: "When you don't get back to normal" 275
Mary: "Ms Busy" 278
Joe: "Joe is stalled" 281
Kevin: "Mr Reactive" 283

Recommended Reading 289
Glossary 293
Index 306

A Note to the Reader

The information in a book like this is necessarily general and may not be directly relevant to your specific circumstances. We are particularly concerned that you not consider this book to be a replacement for your physician and your individual care as a cardiac patient. *Your physician will manage your care.* If you have *any* concerns, including anything you read about in this book that you wish to have clarified, consult with your physician.

Acknowledgments

This book is the product of the confluence of two paths. We first worked together in 1985, when we conducted a systematic evaluation of the emotional states of patients who had survived a near-death event. This joint effort launched our collaboration in the clinical and research fields, in the broad area of cardiac psychiatry and behavioral cardiology, a collaboration that has been assisted greatly by numerous colleagues who have worked with us on various projects over the years. We are particularly grateful for the contributions of Dr David Newman, from cardiology, and Dr Jane Irvine, from psychology. Nadia Woloshyn, an occupational therapist, has treated scores of cardiac patients over the years who are much indebted to her for the individual attention she provided them. Dr Alan Abelsohn has empathically treated the families of many cardiac patients and Sabrina Baker has ably conducted assertiveness groups, for which we owe them a debt of gratitude.

Large numbers of colleagues and friends—too many to mention by name—have helped us over the years to develop expertise in cardiac psychiatry by referring patients, by treating them and by working with us on projects. We gratefully acknowledge their collaboration. We have had the good fortune to work with many outstanding research nurses and research assistants—in particular, Jan Mitchell, Mary Greene, Miney Paquette, Robert Gelaznikas, Janet Edwards, Andrea Snihura and Rima Hosn—without whose dedication our research studies would not have been possible. We also appreciate having been able to collaborate with Dr Terence Kavanagh and Dr Larry Hamm, and the staff and patients at the Toronto Rehabilitation Centre, Cardiac Department.

This book was conceived some years ago, inspired by the obvious lack of heart/mind literature for the cardiac patient. The idea for the book is our own, but it grew out of our interest and involvement in research and theory on cardiology and psychosomatic medicine. Specifically, we were influenced by an article on the psychological rehabilitation of the patient after myocardial infarction (heart attack) by the Wiklund group in 1985. We have integrated our clinical experience with the theory, and what appears here is an amalgam for which we alone can take responsibility.

However, many people have been involved in the preparation of this book. The conception and development occurred with the advice of Rick Gallop and Doug Pepper. Early drafts of portions of this work were reviewed by Cherie Zabow, Dr Shaun Goodman and Nadia Woloshyn, and their input is much appreciated. We are forever grateful to the immense secretarial assistance given by Kim Dawdy and Deborah Bader. Dr Alan Richter has helped in an advisory capacity, and the comments of Dr Shahe Kazarian, Dr Paul Sandor and Dr Colin Shapiro have been valuable. We thank Gary Kaye, our editor Tanya Trafford and our lawyer Marian Hebb. We also acknowledge the personal account of "heart and mind" by one of our patients.

In addition to our gratitude, our patients deserve credit for having contributed to a new focus at the cusp of the specialties, which we believe will become part of the "new medicine" in the twenty-first century.

Finally, without the inspiration of our parents and the unwavering support and encouragement of our families, none of this would have been possible. They alone know how important their encouragement and steadfastness are to us.

Brian Baker
Paul Dorian

Foreword

Heart disease and stroke claim more lives in Canada than any other cause of death. Although great strides have been made over the last number of years, these diseases continue to cost the Canadian economy more than $18 billion per year.

For more than forty years, the Heart and Stroke Foundation has been dedicated to research and education toward reducing death and disability from heart disease and stroke in Canada. Although the death rates remain unacceptably high, research and education are paying off. Since 1955, the death rates due to heart disease and stroke have declined by half, and more and more people each year are surviving cardiac events. This trend places greater demands on the Heart and Stroke Foundation to address the needs of heart attack survivors and their families. Increasingly, the Foundation receives requests from cardiac patients and their families for guidance in their recovery and in managing their lifestyle following a heart attack.

We are delighted to add this volume by Drs Baker and Dorian to our selection of patient education materials. This is our first full-length consumer publication targeting the needs of heart attack survivors and their families. The information in this book is an interesting combination of medical knowledge, medical experience and cardiac patient histories. This allows you to consider this issue from both a medical and a psychological perspective. Drs Baker and Dorian have consolidated their many years of medical practice and experience counseling patients to provide you with this informative insight into heart attack recovery.

As you progress through the book, you will meet six interesting patients, each with unique circumstances affecting their lives following their cardiac events. You will have the opportunity to eavesdrop on their patient–doctor conferences and discussions with family and friends. You will be included as Drs Baker and Dorian confer and exchange medical information with consulting specialists. We are certain you will find these perspectives interesting and relevant.

Most importantly, *Recovering from Heart Disease in Body & Mind* will help you develop a significant understanding of an element of heart disease that is very seldom described—the emotional and psychological aspect of heart attack recovery from the point of view of cardiac patients and their families.

This book is intended to provide you and your family with the insight into the broad impact of heart disease, as well as identifying issues that you might wish to discuss in greater detail with *your* health-care team. Of course, we also hope it will support you and your family as you learn to cope with your personal circumstances and experience with the disease.

On behalf of all of us at the Heart and Stroke Foundation, thank you for your support and for adding *Recovering from Heart Disease in Body & Mind* to your home library. Good luck as you or your loved one begin or continue on the road to recovery. Your success at confronting this disease will support our efforts to greatly reduce death and disability from heart disease and stroke.

Bretta Maloff, M.Ed., R.D.
Heart and Stroke Foundation of Canada

CHAPTER I

Preparing for the Journey: About This Book and How to Use It

The scouts' motto is founded on my initials, it is:
Be prepared, *which means, you are always to be in a state of readiness in mind and body to do your duty.*

—Robert Baden-Powell, *Scouting for Boys* (1908)

WHY DID WE WRITE THIS BOOK?

Coronary heart disease is the most common serious medical disorder in North America. Most people on this continent have a relative or a friend who has suffered from some form of coronary heart disease, and concerns about its causes and consequences are pervasive in the North American consciousness. Mention "heart attack," "bypass surgery," "cholesterol," "exercise," or "stress," and most people will have read or heard much on the subject. There is a huge array of printed information, including books and magazine articles, as well as films and videos and other materials, aimed at educating patients and their families, or simply those possibly at risk for developing heart disease. Organizations such as the Heart and Stroke Foundation of Canada and the American Heart Association, and many authors, including physicians, scientists, nutritionists, exercise advocates and scientific reporters, have added their voices to the swelling commentary on heart disease.

What have we to add to what has already been said and written? As two physicians who, for many years, have been engaged in the care of patients with heart disease and in the scientific exploration of how the mind and the heart interact during their recovery process after cardiac events, we offer a new perspective on the subject. One of us is a psychiatrist with a special interest in the emotional aspects of cardiac disorders, and the other is a cardiologist with expertise in heart rhythm disturbances who has been interested in the scientific study of how the emotional state of patients who have heart attacks and other cardiac problems relates to their recovery.

Over the years, we've noted that much of the information made available to patients and their loved ones has a particular primary perspective: either biological or psychological. Although both of these perspectives are important and valid, we feel that understanding the complicated medical, emotional and social issues surrounding recovery from cardiac events requires a more broadly based point of view—namely, a perspective on the heart and mind that views them as inseparable, intertwined entities that, in effect, function as one.

Since we are both working scientists engaged daily in the use of the scientific method, we have tried where possible to base our thoughts and observations on scientific studies of patients recovering from heart attack and other cardiac illness, rather than relying only on our experiences. Although such experiences, personal and clinical, can be enormously instructive and useful, we feel that the complex, subtle and fascinating relationship between the heart and the mind can properly be the subject of traditional scientific inquiry, and it is in this spirit that we approached the writing of this book.

WHO IS OUR INTENDED READER?

WE HOPE THAT THIS book will be of interest to patients and the loved ones of patients who have been diagnosed with some form of *coronary artery disease*; this group includes those who have had a "heart attack" (known as *myocardial infarction*) or "hardening of the arteries" (*coronary artery disease*) or some sort of event such as *unstable angina* (upper-body discomfort experienced at rest or for a prolonged period) and those who have had a cardiac procedure such as *angioplasty* (balloon dilatation of coronary arteries) or coronary artery bypass surgery. We explain all these terms in more detail as we go along (and in the glossary). We have avoided using too many abbreviations, but for the sake of convenience shorten "coronary artery disease" to *CAD*, and "CAD event" or "CAD outcome" to *cardiac event* or *cardiac outcome*. The term *patient* has a clinical, antiseptic ring to it, but we use it in this book to signify the person who is the subject under discussion, who will have experienced a cardiac event. As there is probably also no single satisfactory word for all those *significant others* of the patient, be they spouse, partner, relative, family, confidante, loved one, caregiver or any interested party, we use these terms interchangeably.

HOW IS THIS BOOK DIFFERENT FROM OTHER BOOKS ON HEART DISEASE?

THERE ARE A NUMBER of books available on heart disease that ably describe the "what" of CAD; that is, they are excellent at giving information on the risks for and treatment of the disease. What they largely ignore, however, is the *experience* of a cardiac event—that is, both the physical and the emotional components in combination. As doctors, we have spent much of our time trying to understand what cardiac patients subjectively go through and feel. As authors, we have tried to identify this experience for you.

It is always a relief to know what is a normal response to a cardiac event. And, if the response is abnormal in some way, the patient and his or her relatives can at least know that benefits can be had from professional advice, and treatment if need be, as all clinical conditions respond to some type of intervention. Often patients and their families feel considerably better once they receive acknowledgment, or validation, that the patient's experience of CAD is normal or expected.

However, we focus on the experience not only to make people *feel* better. Recent research has shown that certain negative emotions may be linked to a less positive cardiac outcome. For that reason, we address how to alleviate these negative emotions, so that the patient will not only feel better, but may be able to lower the likelihood of recurring events as well.

Once an event resulting from coronary artery disease occurs, a "journey" begins that will take weeks, months, or even a year or more to complete. This journey comprises a series of stages, or *phases.* If you do not recognize the landmarks along the way, you are liable to get lost. In this book, we show you the way on the journey to recovery, but we also keep in mind that each person, like his or her fingerprint, is unique, and embarks with a particular history, social circle and medical status.

This book is divided into two parts: "The Guide" and "Directions." The first section describes the path from "Event," through "Aftermath," "Recuperation" and "Rehabilitation," to "Recovery" to help patients and their loved ones identify what they are going through and understand whether what they are feeling is normal or unusual, and to suggest what can be done during each of these phases.

Everybody wants to know what they must *do* to get better. Patients are understandably very motivated to learn what they can about how to improve their outcome after an event like a heart attack—especially soon after it. Those who wish to obtain detailed information and guidelines will find what they need in Part Two, "Directions." Here, unlike the majority of books that discuss this aspect of recovery after a cardiac event, this book does not set out any hard and fast rules about "programs" for you to follow. The truth is that, for many patients, programs are difficult to stick with, since so much of the ability to change and adapt is dependent on *where* you are on the path to recovery. For this reason, we have tailored our suggested activities to the appropriate stages of your journey, and thus to your readiness to undertake them.

As well, this book is different from most in that it takes an integrated approach to recovery, focusing on both "heart" and "mind." Thus, Part One discusses the signposts on the journey from event to recovery in terms of both the physical and the emotional; Part Two provides detailed discussions of key issues—of the heart and the mind—for those who have had experience of heart disease. As well, you will find dialogues called "Heart to Mind." In these, we speak to you in our separate voices of "Heart" and "Mind" about three key aspects of the journey to recovery: "The Third Way," "Themes of Healing" and "Ready for Rehabilitation."

We have evolved a motif for this book—"Heart to Heart"—by which we mean "frank, intimate and sincere." First, we attempt to be as direct as possible, within the constraints of writing for an unknown reader. That means we are often forced to be general, rather than specific, about some topics in this book, and we ask that you collaborate with us by concentrating on those statements that best relate to your particular circumstances. We wish to emphasize that these general statements are grounded in our own and others' research and, most importantly, in conclusions drawn from our own clinical experience.

As specialists, we are only too aware that each individual is unique, and that describing the emotional experience of CAD in general terms is particularly problematic. The emotional response to a cardiac event is very subjective, and very particular, and what one goes through can be almost sacred in that one's life has changed. Nonetheless, our regular contact with many cardiac patients has led us to an understanding that distinct general themes emerge from these very particular experiences, and we confidently share these with you.

Second, we are talking to *you*, patient and loved one, and sharing with you open discussion between us (the authors), six patients who are on the journey to recovery, and their loved ones. These roundtable discussions, called "Forum," appear after each of the stages of the journey discussed in Part One, and the outcomes for the "Select Six"—representing the integration of Heart and Mind on the journey to recovery—are outlined in Part Two.

Before you turn to Part One, we offer you our first "Heart to Mind." In it we introduce ourselves and sum up briefly why we wrote this book.

DR BAKER: When I was doing my specialist's training, I was intrigued by how the family affects the course of illness. Later, as a psychiatrist, when Dr Dorian started to send me referrals of patients who had suffered life-threatening cardiac events, I became more familiar with the situations and problems of cardiac patients in general, and looked at ways to help them and their families. I am particularly taken with the way the mind responds to the impact of an event like heart attack, or even a procedure such as bypass surgery. I have noticed that when certain patterns are identified, patients and their families seem to appreciate knowing about them, and this makes treatment easier. Patients attending rehabilitation programs—especially patients who do not have any overt emotional problems—are able to identify with a phased approach to emotional recovery after a cardiac event. I am always being asked to recommend appropriate literature for patient and family, and was only too aware that no material for both patient and family that was useful as a guide from event to recovery was available.

DR DORIAN: I am a cardiologist who started my professional life interested in research on disorders of heart rhythm. I continue to practice cardiology with a special interest in these "electrical" disturbances of the heart. However, early in my career, I noticed that the psychological elements of heart disease were not considered to be very important by most cardiologists. I had the opportunity to collaborate with Dr Baker in the treatment of patients with both psychological symptoms and heart disease, and became rapidly convinced that patients' attitudes, beliefs and social circumstances had a very important influence in the consequences of their heart disease, especially on their quality of life.

Patients and families have many unanswered questions regarding their medical illness and how best to cope with the emotional consequences. Very few books or materials are available that discuss both what is happening to the heart and the relationship between the emotions and the heart.

DR BAKER: Our hope is that we will address those needs and contribute toward a meaningful recovery for both patient and family.

PART ONE:

The Guide

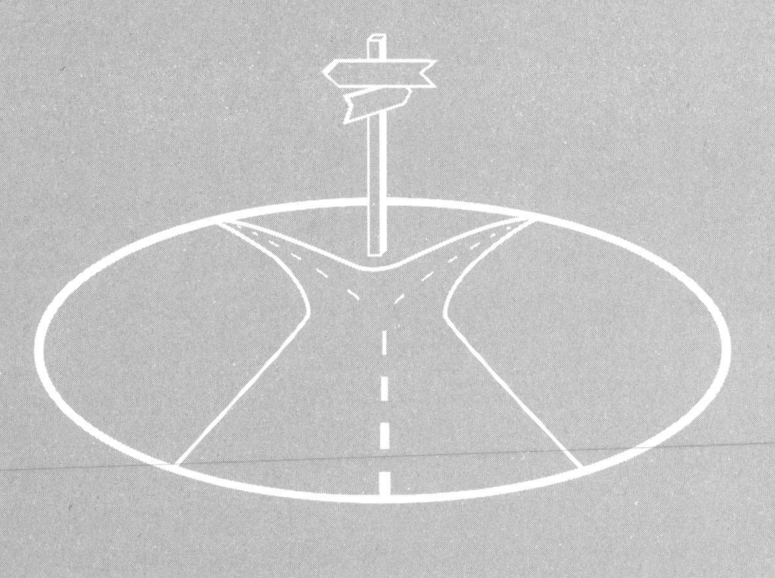

CHAPTER 2

Guide to the Journey: An Introduction

journey 1. act of going from one place to another, especially at a long distance 2. time taken for this

—Oxford Dictionary of Current English

WHAT YOU NEED TO KNOW ABOUT "THE GUIDE"

The response to a cardiac event develops in phases and can be seen in terms of the metaphor of a journey. Although there are myriad ways for the phases to present themselves, both in their characteristics and in their duration, the sequence in which they occur is quite predictable. Typically, there are five phases, although some of them overlap, and each has its own medical (cardiac) and emotional aspects. In addition, each triggers fairly typical responses in the patient's significant others, especially the closest ones. Responses of the loved ones can be expected to be less marked or prolonged, but sometimes can be even more pronounced than the patient's.

In Chapters 3 to 7, we discuss the five phases of your journey to recovery. Here we summarize them for you, to provide an overview of that journey.

Event

The first phase, the event, comprises the cardiac event itself and the lead-up to it. In essence, this phase has to do with two versions of the question "*What happened?*" In the first case, the question is meant in a literal way: "What in fact happened?" The response to this question is that an event occurred, signifying CAD. Therefore, Chapter 3 reviews CAD in brief, keeping in mind that too much detail may be confusing, particularly in light of the second version of the question. In this case, the question is being asked as more of an outcry: "What happened?!" This emotionally charged question signifies the initial emotional response to what has actually been a threat to the patient. What now happens to protect the individual from having to deal with the full emotional impact of this threat is a type of emotional numbing that is termed "shock."

Aftermath

The second phase, the aftermath, is actually the tail end of the preceding phase, but it is distinctive enough to warrant discussion as separate. Chapter 4 helps you understand "where you are" after the event, which is particularly important at a time when hospitalization of only a few days has become the norm. Medically, active treatment in the form of medications, and individual and family instruction, as well as early steps towards rehabilitation, have already been started and, before you know it, you are back home and expected to follow through on these aspects of treatment. It is important for you, your family and your managing professionals to realize that, emotionally, a lot has occurred in a short space of time, and that a journey has begun that can take up to a year and beyond to complete. At this time, the patient can feel somewhat lost and emotionally disoriented, and this response can coincide with what can be the most difficult time for the loved ones, often marked by a period of "overwatchfulness" (or "hypervigilance") that can be harmful and upsetting for everyone involved.

Recuperation

The third phase is recuperation. As the body heals, medical evaluation and treatment proceed, often punctuated by commonly performed procedures such as angioplasty or bypass surgery. The main aspects of tests, procedures and medications are briefly reviewed in Chapter 5, and it is particularly in relation to these that the reader will benefit from referring to Part Two, "Directions," if more detail is required. Distinct from the healing of the body, there is now a release of emotional energies, which had been suppressed during the shock of the event. It is important for those patients and their loved ones who are going through this release to recognize that emotional reaction during this particular period makes them vulnerable. As reassurance, we describe what is the "normal" experience during this phase. Four common emotional reactions are highlighted—anxiety, sadness, low mood and anger. Each one has its context and explanation. Here it will be important to understand when seeking professional advice is advisable. Typical "imbalances" are described, including the vicious cycle of physical symptoms and anxiety, the symptom constellation of clinical depression, as well as potential upsets in the family system. As recuperation advances, a balance is sought by both mind and body, and in the family system, preparing, as it were, for the next phase.

Rehabilitation

We know that rehabilitation, in the cardiac sense, commences, for many, during hospitalization. We use the term "rehabilitation" in a broad sense, to describe a period of consistent structured activity, when up to 80 percent of those who have had a cardiac event will be eligible for the types of supervised community programs that have been so successful in improving quality of life in CAD patients. This phase, unlike those preceding it, has a harmonious emotional component, which has been termed "reconstruction." In Chapter 6, we emphasize the importance of adaptive denial and the avoidance of the sick role. We review the cardinal feature of this phase—the programs—and, here too, readers who wish to know more details, including relaxation techniques and anger management, can consult Part Two, "Directions."

Recovery

The term "recovery" is controversial, at least for cardiologists, given the recognition that one does not "recover" from CAD *per se*. It is for that reason we distinguish between CAD and the *event* of heart disease, as one can clearly recover from the event, both physically and emotionally. As we point out in Chapter 7, to deal with the ongoing nature of CAD, it is important for patients and their loved ones to be realistic. Also we highlight the challenge of maintenance, a problem that should be neither neglected nor minimized. We support the notion of developing "pleasurable heart-healthy habits," something that has proved valuable to many who became discouraged when they thought all the work had been done, only to be reminded that still more was expected of them.

While the journey will be hard at times, its benefits are numerous. As you progress toward recovery, the gains you make during each phase—in particular, self-effectiveness—will carry you to the next of life's journeys prepared.

Meet Tony

Tony is one of our "Select Six"—the six patients we have chosen to represent those recovering from a cardiac event. You will meet the other five patients in subsequent chapters of the Guide, and they will become equally familiar to you, especially after you have heard some of what they and their loved ones have to say in our roundtable discussion—"Forum"—at the end of each chapter. (To know more about what happened to each of the six patients, who illustrate different ways of dealing with the cardiac event, read "Six Journeys," in Part Two.)

The "Select Six" are composites, based on actual case histories of patients we have managed in our clinical cardiology and cardiac psychiatry practices. Readers need to understand that these "patients," while representative, do not define a particular course that *must* be followed. Rather, they are used to illustrate trends with which many, but not all, will identify. These patients will help *you* identify where you and your significant other are on your journey, and guide you from the event toward a good recovery.

FORUM (TONY): Does awareness help?

Tony is a fifty-four-year-old man, employed in the parts department of a hardware store. He is married, with a twenty-year-old son, who has left home. About a year ago, Tony had a heart attack, from which he suffered no complications; a week later, he was discharged from the hospital. He attended a rehabilitation program at the local hospital but stopped it after four months because he was "too busy." He is now seeing a cardiologist at regular intervals and is receiving cardiac medications, although he frequently forgets to take his pills. He is able to work. If he moves quickly when walking his dog or if he lifts heavy objects at work, he experiences chest pain. He stopped smoking after his heart attack but about six months ago gradually began to smoke again. He is very fond of meat and hasn't really changed his diet very much since the event.

We invited Tony and his wife to review this book to see if they could identify with what we had written and to participate in this, our first "Forum," a discussion between "the patient," his significant other, and us (Dr Baker and Dr Dorian).

WIFE: We were very pleased that you allowed us to look at your manuscript.

TONY: You mean *you* were interested in reading it!

DR BAKER: Tony, are you implying that you are not sure whether this could help you?

TONY: This stuff may be interesting, doc, but I really don't see how this has to do with me. I don't get all this about "the mind and the heart." I am just trying to get along, to do my work, and live with my heart disease, that's all.

WIFE: I am not so sure that he is doing as well as he thinks.

TONY: What do you mean?

WIFE: Well, you seem to be coughing and a bit short of breath. You haven't been too interested in going out to see our friends, although I notice you sneaking out to the back deck to smoke cigarettes almost every day now.

TONY: I don't think I'm too bad. It's true I get chest pain every so often, but that's only when I push myself.

WIFE: Yes, like when you walk the dog, and what about when we want to make love?

TONY: Are you saying you are unhappy with me?

WIFE: Of course not. I'm just not one to bury my head in the sand.

DR BAKER: There seem to be issues about Tony's health, and between the two of you. Let's begin by asking whether either of you found any points we made to be valuable. Maybe we can start with just after the heart attack.

WIFE: Well, Tony's not one to dwell on things. He was fine in the hospital, but it was me that was having to understand what happened. The difficult time was when he came home. I was worried about him.

TONY: I'm not one to fret about things, but I was at a loose end in those first few weeks when I had nothing much to do.

WIFE: Things settled down once he could get busy. When he got back to work and joined that rehab program, he was more of himself. Even now, though, he still doesn't seem totally well.

TONY: I guess I haven't been leading as normal a life as I could and as I would like. Are you suggesting that my attitude can affect my heart?

DR DORIAN: That is exactly what we are suggesting, Tony. Not only can having chest pain limit your activities, but your outlook on life, as well as what you do, such as your smoking habit, can directly influence how much chest pain you have. For example, if you were to work with your doctors to make a commitment to taking your medications consistently, to stop smoking and to be positive about the future, you would be surprised at how much better you would feel.

TONY: Well, of course I *would like* to stop smoking, to exercise and to improve my diet. I just slipped, I suppose. I was interested in what you wrote about having healthy habits that are enjoyable, and I should read that again, because the problem is: I like to do things that are *not* good for me. I guess if I'd known more, I could have been helped, like my wife said, right after the heart attack, when I wasn't quite sure what was happening, and also now, when I am *supposed* to be doing all these healthy things.

DR BAKER: I don't want Tony to think that he is being ganged up on. As long as you follow your program, we know that there is some good in *not* unduly worrying about things. From this discussion, though, it seems there are many areas that could be explored which could help both of you a fair amount. I have to admit that you do present a challenge to us.

TONY: Why's that?

DR BAKER: Well, most of us believe that knowing about your condition, generally, is a good thing, especially if it leads to being aware of your self. This is all the more so when it comes to something that has been a threat to you, such as the heart attack. It is difficult to deal with what is going on, in those early days and weeks afterwards. That is why we have talked about the phases that one goes through. You deal with things differently, over time. The same point applies to the loved ones, who also go through this recovery process. In your case, it seems that it was "the wife" and not "the patient" who was more directly affected. I say "directly" because I know that you *were* affected as well, Tony.

The last point I wanted to make was about *now.* The past is one thing, but it does seem like there are current issues to be dealt with. By this I mean, staying healthy, by managing your smoking, eating and exercise, maybe your sexual relations too. My only concern is that you will feel bombarded with all this information, Tony.

TONY: No, it feels good to learn that I can improve my health. Maybe I should read the manuscript again and let all this sink in before I can go on to the next step, whatever that is!

Dr Baker: Tony is raising a key point: How do we motivate people? Trying to insist on something doesn't always work well. I have found that the more forcefully we make our arguments, the more the person backs off.

Dr Dorian: Motivation has to come from within. Doctors and caregivers cannot really compel or "push" patients to change. We can only point out the strategies patients can use to help them alter their attitudes and behavior. The first and crucial step is to *want* to change. I don't mean idle, offhand wishes, but a true committed desire that accepts the challenges ahead. This commitment requires thought and preparation, and is a specific step unto itself, not a "given" in preparing for change.

Wife: Well, I've found it helpful to read about this, and to discuss it.

Dr Baker: We were hoping that the Forum could serve the purpose of going over a theme of each chapter, and could be used as a springboard for discussion. The theme here is how being aware of one's condition can help to motivate you to a better recovery.

Last word, Tony?

Tony: Well, I have started to know more; now I must *do* more.

CHAPTER 3

Event

***event** 1. thing that happens 2. fact of a thing's occurring*

—Oxford Dictionary of Current English

An event has happened, upon which it is difficult to speak, and impossible to be silent.

—Edmund Burke

What's wrong with Anna?

Anna was finding it hard to concentrate. She was sitting in the movie theater and becoming increasingly aware of discomfort in her chest. Her husband glanced at her. As the ache became established, Anna tried to calm herself: "Is this a run-of-the-mill angina attack? It's been only a couple of months since my heart attack. They had said it was only 'mild.' What is going on now?"

An hour later, Anna lay in the intensive care unit. Time had seemed distorted, even as she was waiting for the ambulance to take her to the emergency room. Now, she was hooked up to various contraptions. She felt strange, somewhat unreal. Last time, she had handled things well; now, frankly, she was a bit scared. Then, she had believed the doctors, and she seemed to be getting better. Now, who knew?

Anna is the second of the six patients whom we have chosen to represent what people go through during and after a cardiac event. The scene described above occurred in the context of a prior heart attack. Anna managed her first episode without too much trouble, but we are not sure how she will cope with it this time. On the one hand, there is "trying to make sense of what is happening"; on the other hand, there is the "alarm" mechanism, whose intensity varies, depending on the individual. As well, the family is going to be affected in a major way, and an extra burden will be placed on the shoulders of the main caregiver, often the spouse. Even though the event and the response to it do not last long, their effect is significant, and they launch a journey that can go on for months, even a year or more. After we have reviewed the Event phase, we'll return to Anna and her husband to see what they have to say, a year after her first admission to hospital, about their particular experiences of the Event.

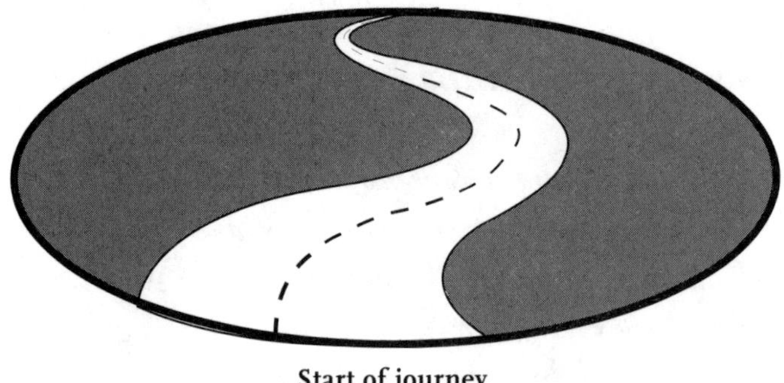

Start of journey

WHAT HAPPENED?

EVEN THOUGH HEART ATTACK is common, the experience of heart attack is anything but commonplace. The same can be said for any cardiac event. What each person goes through is an experience special to him or her, and no amount of dramatizing is necessary to underscore this fact. How the event is directly experienced by each individual will vary widely. One way of understanding what happens is to say that patients who have suffered a cardiac event ask two questions of crucial, and interrelated, importance. The words are the same, but you can appreciate the difference by saying them out aloud.

The first is articulated in a calm, measured way. Now, say this slowly: "*What . . . happened?*"

Expressed this way, the question means: What, *in fact*, happened? The questioner is asking for information, and the response is that an event requiring immediate attention, and signifying CAD, has occurred. We will answer this query in a moment.

For the next rendition of the question, imagine you are in California and have just noticed the floors and walls and bed shaking. Now, say this with full resonance, and dramatic effect: "*WHAT HAPPENED?!*"

Expressed this way, the question means that a threat has occurred and an emotional alarm has been sounded. This completely different version of the question is likely processed by a separate part of the brain—the limbic system, or emotional brain.

This exercise is an exaggeration of how an individual tries to deal with a cardiac event: by attempting to make sense of what has just happened *and* by reacting emotionally.

Making intellectual sense of the meaning of the symptoms usually starts right away. The experience of chest pain or tightness or shortness of breath leads to an emergency hospital visit and immediate treatment. Most patients are made aware, if they are not already, that they are having cardiac symptoms and may be in the throes of a heart attack.

Making emotional sense of what has happened takes more time. This phase is especially confusing since the actual events are still unfolding, and the seriousness of the attack, its short- and long-term consequences and the treatments required are not clear right now, or even predictable. It's a lot like longing to know how a thriller ends after reading the exciting introduction—only the patient can't turn to the end of the book to find out what happened. The patient has to live through the story first.

By way of introduction to the event that launches the journey, we must remind our readers and their loved ones that CAD outcome has changed markedly for the better in recent years. Things are somewhat confusing during the event itself. After the event, a process of healing will take place, and will provide the time and the peace of mind necessary for the situation to become clearer.

WHAT, IN FACT, HAPPENED TO MY HEART?

THE MOST DRAMATIC of acute heart events is a "heart attack," known as a *myocardial infarction* (MI). This term refers to permanent damage to the heart caused by interruption in blood flow to the heart muscle itself, resulting in loss of heart muscle and its replacement by scar. The heart is a muscle like any other muscle in the body; in order to pump effectively, it must receive oxygen; this is delivered by blood vessels that run across the outer surface of the heart and are known as the coronary arteries. Much like the structure of a tree, large coronary arteries, which represent the trunks of a branching arterial system, divide into major branches that run on the outer surface of the heart, and then divide into many smaller branches, and ultimately into small "twigs," which supply blood and oxygen to the heart muscle cells themselves. Not surprisingly, if any of these large trunks or branches become obstructed or blocked, blood cannot flow, and the portion of heart muscle that normally receives blood and oxygen through these branches will suffer permanent damage. If such permanent damage occurs, it is called a heart attack.

Almost all patients who have heart attacks do so because they have *coronary atherosclerosis*, or hardening of the arteries to the heart, which is a very slowly evolving process, taking many decades, resulting in a buildup of cholesterol, calcium and scar tissue on the inside of an artery, gradually choking off its blood supply. In response to this *injury* inside the blood vessel itself, the body may respond by producing a blood clot; this can be the "last straw," resulting in the sudden blockage of an artery that has been already narrowed by the "atherosclerotic" (hardening) process. If such a blood clot forms, the muscle cells downstream from the narrowing and acute blockage (*occlusion*) fail to receive enough blood, and the consequence is one or more of: chest discomfort, tightness, pain, shortness of breath or nausea, otherwise known as *myocardial ischemia* (lack of enough blood to the heart). If this clot spontaneously dissolves or is promptly treated and dissolves, a heart attack may not actually occur, but the threat of heart attack prompts hospitalization, investigation, and often treatment. If blood flow is interrupted for a sufficiently long period of time, permanent damage to the heart muscle cells can occur.

Many patients with "hardening of the arteries" have chest discomfort or shortness of breath when they are active. This is known as *angina*, and it results from an increased need for oxygen by the exercising heart muscle that cannot be supplied by the narrowed artery. This is analogous to what occurs when several lanes of a highway are blocked by construction—off-peak traffic can flow almost normally, but the increased flow of traffic during rush hour creates major traffic jams. Such patients have symptoms during physical or emotional stress, but these subside with rest. A predictable pattern of chest discomfort with activity, and which subsides with rest, is known as *stable angina*.

A heart attack or *unstable angina* is suspected when pain occurs at rest or without provocation. A "heart attack" is the result of complete blockage of an artery, which leads to irreversible heart damage. This damage may be very minor or more severe, depending on the size of the artery and the amount of muscle that it supplies, and the period of time it is blocked. Administering a "clot buster," or *thrombolytic agent*, early after the onset of pain can considerably limit heart damage. It is this opportunity to treat patients early—often expressed by cardiologists with the saying "Time is muscle"—that makes it very important for patients to understand the warning signs of a heart attack and to consult a doctor or go to an emergency room immediately rather than waiting.

Unstable angina is a warning from the heart, a "yellow light," that there is fairly major shortage of blood flow, but fortunately it produces minimal to no permanent damage. The signal the heart is sending out is that the narrowing is fairly severe, often temporary and due to a blood clot that significantly but not completely blocks blood flow. Medications and bed rest can lead to these clots dissolving and the situation returning to the status quo, or the blockage may become more severe but still not complete. Patients with unstable angina can be treated and spared future heart events, with no heart damage having been done.

With either a heart attack or unstable angina, patients are invariably admitted to a hospital, usually to a *coronary care unit* (CCU—a type of intensive care unit where there is close and continuous nursing and medical supervision) and are treated with medications to dissolve clots in the arteries, prevent further clotting and reduce the work of the heart. Sometimes, attempts are made to immediately "open up" the blocked artery using tubes and balloons inserted directly into the heart's arteries, a procedure known as *balloon angioplasty*. Rarely, emergency *bypass surgery* may be performed.

During the hospital stay, patients receive drug therapy, stabilization and treatment of any complications that may occur.

Fortunately, over 90 percent of patients admitted to hospitals with acute heart attacks survive without major complications, and often are hospitalized for only five to seven days. During the initial period, there will not be any major tests in most instances, but patients are treated, closely monitored and stabilized. Prior to discharge from the hospital, a patient may undergo tests to assess the potential risk for a repeat heart attack or future serious heart events. These tests often include an ultrasound of the heart (*echocardiogram*), an exercise test or X-ray imaging of the blood flow to the heart (*thallium* or *Cardiolite® imaging*), and sometimes *coronary angiography* (an X ray of the blood vessels to the heart). These tests are discussed in detail in Part Two of this book.

WHAT HAPPENED TO ME?!

TRYING TO EXPLAIN a subjective experience is a difficult thing—particularly when the event that triggers it may be very dramatic. There is so much variation that we can only highlight some common characteristics. Perhaps the clearest way to present this is through a series of figures. Figure 3.1 shows one's experience (the

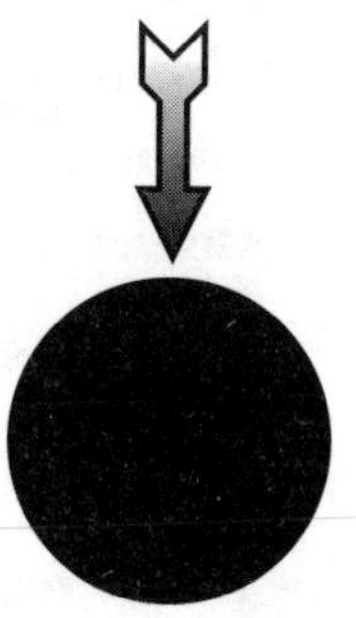

Fig. 3.1

Experiencing the event

circle) and the event (the downward-pointing arrow above the circle). Simple! However, we must keep in mind that the way each of us processes events—that is, the way each of us experiences the happenings of the world—is unique. Not only are the details of the response subtly or greatly different between people, but the *intensity* of response varies from ultracool to very dramatic, with most of us in the middle, as well as the *timing* of response, from immediate to delayed.

In figure 3.2 we see that the arrow (or event) has now penetrated the circle. It has crossed the boundary, gone into our consciousness; this is what we call the *impact* of the event. Now, although there is a wide variation in people's emotional responses, there *are* common features. Generally, our response is one of alarm, but on the surface, it is dulled or muted even though, below the surface, an emotional upheaval may be taking place. The term coined by the crisis theorists for this phenomenon—*shock*—has a dramatic connotation.

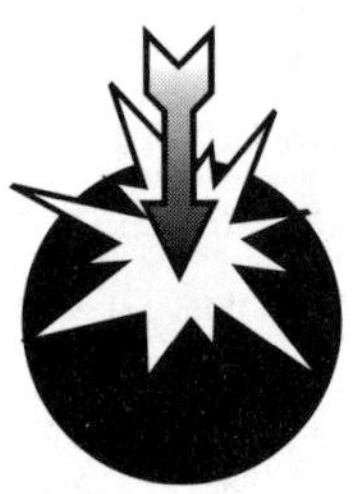

Fig. 3.2
Impact of event

The outward calmness shown by most patients can be surprising both to them and to their loved ones. Although this self-protective mechanism belies the suppressed emotions under the surface, it helps deal with the surprise and fear of the event itself. A potential problem can be that loved ones fail to understand that "things may not be okay even though everything looks okay."

The shock response diverts attention from what is actually going on—a potentially serious cardiac event. While the body is being worked on, so to speak, the mind shuts down. This is similar to being given a local anesthetic; say, for example when we are receiving stitches for a deep cut. We are protected from feeling what is being done to us. On a psychological level, a type of *numbing* is occurring. This is illustrated in figure 3.3, where a separate area representing this emotional numbing has been cordoned off, in response to the event.

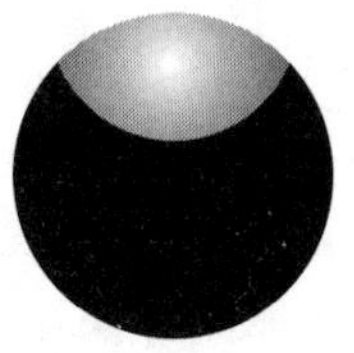

Fig. 3.3
Emotional Numbing

The shock response corresponds to the time surrounding the event; this means the onset, the lead-up and the admission to a hospital and, often, the early discharge period. One of the reasons for shock to persist on arrival home may have something to do with the current practice of releasing patients with relatively uncomplicated cardiac events after only a few days of hospitalization.

So, the duration for the shock response is relatively short, depending on what has happened and how we process this event. It may last only hours, and it is usually over in a matter of days. For some, though, it can go on for weeks. In such cases, the patient has not only been distressed by the event, but has experienced something *more*. This "something more" is what we call a *post-traumatic* response. In these cases, there is often an extra component to the story, as the case history on the next page illustrates. However, for most patients, the shock response is a brief one, very brief compared to the rest of the journey of recovery.

It is not uncommon for *repeated cardiac events* to affect the shock response (see Anna, page 32). In group sessions at the rehabilitation program, there may be a person who volunteers that he cannot relate to the various experiences in the journey to recovery. At the same time, there will be someone else who identifies easily with these phases. This second person will have coped famously with a first episode, but a second episode will intensify his or her identification with the experiences we discuss. There is not necessarily anything abnormal about the response of the first individual. Nobody prescribes how you must feel.

Another possibility is that the shock is pronounced the first time, especially when the event comes out of the blue, as it so often does, but is diminished in a repeat episode. Predicting how the human mind will respond is a hazardous activity.

Sometimes the shock can be unusually *prolonged*. Dr Baker once saw a woman who, a few weeks back, had had a heart attack, but her recovery had been unusually slow and the cardiologist wanted an opinion. Initially, not much information could be obtained that would unlock the problem. After probing the question of her fatigue for signs of possible depression, suddenly there was an outpouring of anger! The story emerged that this woman was very unhappy with her husband, to whom she had been married for twenty-five years. While he was apparently committed to staying in the marriage, he was unable to show love and express caring for her. She had complained to him about this, which had made the situation worse. (Harriet Lerner elegantly describes this common "pursuer–distancer" interaction in her book *The Dance of Anger*.)

When this woman's chest pain started, she had asked her husband to take her to the hospital, but he had refused, implying that there was no basis to her complaints. Her adult children were finally contacted and took her to the emergency room, and it was discovered that the delay had worsened her condition. This left her in an extended shock phase, which was finally resolved with the emergence of anger toward her spouse. This experience amounted to a traumatic one for this woman, and she therefore had features of a post-traumatic response. Most patients do not have such a pronounced response to a cardiac event, the shock usually lasting, as mentioned, hours or days. Shock itself can be an "unreal," anxious and confusing state that quickly merges with your experience in the aftermath, the subject of the next chapter.

WHAT TO EXPECT

GENERALLY, PATIENTS SPEND the first one to three days in the hospital in a *coronary care unit*, where they receive intensive nursing care and continuous monitoring of the *electrocardiogram* (ECG). Subsequent convalescence is generally on an "ordinary" cardiac ward, although close observation and ECG monitoring are often maintained.

Most patients have a fairly prompt resolution of their chest pains and other symptoms when they are admitted to a hospital and treated. In a few cases, symptoms continue and require immediate investigation. However, most patients do feel "stunned," fatigued and out of sorts during this time. Such feelings are prompted in part by the major changes to the heart and the body caused by the event itself; the treatments, which often have minor but unpleasant side effects; and the tests, which can cause some anxiety. Do not be surprised if your doctors are unable to give you a clear picture of the future, since the intermediate and long-term outcomes cannot be clearly predicted during the first few days after a cardiac event. (We describe the various tests doctors can do to help predict the long-term outcome, and the various treatments patients may receive to improve their well-being and future prospects, in Part Two, pages 162–179.)

During the event, the mind is protected by the shock response. As long as the shock doesn't intrude on treatment, it may even be helpful. So, the first piece of advice is simply to follow the instructions on how to deal with an event as it is declaring itself (see "Emergency," pages 158–159) and if you feel distant, spacy, confused, with varying degrees of strong emotions—don't panic! It is important to recognize that this is the shock response and that usually it will fade quite quickly. In most cases, this fading will start once you are in the protective world of the coronary care unit, and your condition is stable—usually within one or two days. With reassurance will come relief; however, this doesn't mean the remainder of the journey will be straightforward.

The *role of the spouse* during an event should not be underestimated. The "significant others" need to be aware not only of what the patient is going through, but also of what they themselves will experience. But, first, a job must be done. This means seeking medical attention immediately. Sometimes an assertive attitude is required to communicate what the problem is and also to determine what in fact has happened. As spouses may be somewhat shocked themselves, they should be prepared to check that they understand what it is that is being said to them. It helps to stay calm. At this time, the executive functions for the families pass to the spouses. They are the interim presidents, whether they like it or not! They need to see that they are in control of themselves and the situation, even if they feel otherwise. Don't worry—the event itself is usually short-lived and although there will be more to deal with, it will probably be of lesser intensity.

FORUM (ANNA): Dealing with the event

Anna is a fifty-eight-year-old businesswoman who runs a busy dry-cleaning operation with her brothers. Anna had been healthy all her life except for easily controlled high blood pressure, and had no inkling of heart disease until a year ago, when she had a mild heart attack. Soon after, she went back to work and was fine until a month later, when, at a movie theater, she began to have chest pain and had to be rushed to a hospital. An angiogram showed she had narrowing of a major artery, and this was successfully treated with balloon angioplasty. Although she had been quite alarmed that the pains had recurred, she again recovered quickly and went back to work.

Anna was surprised and puzzled that a few weeks later she experienced heaviness in the chest and an odd feeling of weakness. This didn't worry her much at first, but it began to happen with mild activities, even taking out the garbage or carrying groceries. Anna did not disclose this and it went on for some time before worsening; this time she had her weakness and heaviness for two hours before going to the hospital. Another recurrence of the blockage was found and again treated with angioplasty. Since then she has remained physically well.

Anna's marriage of thirty years has gone through its ups and downs. Over the years she and her husband became somewhat distant from each other, even though they used to be close.

We asked Anna and her husband to review this chapter a year after her initial hospitalization, and they join us for this Forum.

ANNA: I certainly would have appreciated reading this after my heart attack, the first time I was in the hospital.

DR BAKER: Why is that?

Anna: Because I didn't know what was to come! I mean, once the doctors had reassured me, I seemed to handle it well that time. I was discharged after, what, a few days? And then I was back home. But it was the *second* time I was hospitalized that I was quite shaken. And when I felt unwell for the *third* time—well, I couldn't get over that! I didn't tell anyone at first. I just walked around being bothered about it.

Dr Baker: It must have been quite a burden for you. People respond very differently during the event. The one may have a strong response; the other, a type of non-response. What *you* are illustrating is something that can happen with people who have recurrent cardiac problems. At the beginning, they can take it in their stride and the shock is over before they know it—in a matter of hours. But, from what you are telling me, when it happened again, you were greatly affected.

Anna: Yes, it seemed that every time I got over an attack and got back on my feet, I would get knocked over again. Each time I had a problem, I said to myself, "Oh no, here we go again!"

Dr Dorian: You know, Anna, it is unfortunately not rare for patients to have recurrences of heart symptoms or heart problems, and there can often seem to be no end to it. Whenever you have a new attack you will be faced with great uncertainties about what is happening and what the future holds. Although your doctors cannot predict the future, they can treat you to help you get over the "hump," so to speak; it is often frustrating to patients not to have all the answers available right away. As in your case, patients often do well in the end, even though they may have had a "bumpy ride."

HUSBAND: I could see that Anna was upset about something. But that's the trouble with you, Anna—you're always brooding about something or other that has upset you when the rest of us have already forgotten about it. How was I supposed to know that you'd been having pains all that time? I'm not a mind reader.

ANNA: There's no need to get sarcastic. Besides, the third time I had to go to the hospital I nearly missed getting my clot-buster treatment.

HUSBAND: I'm sorry. I didn't mean to come across like that, but you can read bad intention into what I say. In this case, I think I know what you are getting at. Can I explain?

ANNA: Go ahead.

HUSBAND: Well, it's like that story of the lady who was angry with her husband when he didn't heed her request to take her pain seriously. The truth is that, before all this heart business, we weren't getting along so well. In fact, our marriage was falling by the wayside, what with Anna so involved in the family business. Then after the heart attack, we thought she was going to be fine. Instead, it turned out to be just one thing after the next.

DR BAKER: It's true that sometimes illness brings people together; at other times, it pushes them apart.

HUSBAND: At the beginning, we got a little closer, as Anna was handling things well. Then, after that second admission, she seemed so troubled. She can be a bitter person, you know, and frankly I started to turn a blind eye to what was going on—so much so, that the last time, it was two hours of continuous problems before I became convinced to take her to the hospital. I still feel badly about the delay in getting her to the hospital that third time, even though Anna says I shouldn't.

DR BAKER: This is not an uncommon scenario. The opposite scenario is also seen—when the couple keeps rushing to the emergency room. For the spouses, the situation is difficult, as they are also having an emotional response and may also feel helpless. Besides remaining calm, which is always advisable, and calling the ambulance, from the medical perspective what can you recommend for the spouse, Dr Dorian?

DR DORIAN: The start of an attack, especially if it is not the first one, is a particularly difficult time for both patient and family. First of all, it is often not clear whether there is a true emergency, or whether the problem is a minor one. If the symptoms are similar to those of the original attack, they should be taken seriously, especially if chest pain or discomfort lasts more than half an hour or so. Sometimes, as in Anna's case, the symptoms are not clearcut and may not be typical "heart symptoms" or may be different from symptoms previously felt. If unusual feelings *persist*, it is always wise to seek professional advice right away.

Once in the hospital, significant others have difficulty coping since they are faced with yet another disruption in their routine, with hospital visits, uncertainty about the present and future, looking after the family affairs, and "holding things together." It is important that no long-term decisions be made at this time, but that the family as well as the patient be "patient" until the fog clears from the acute event.

ANNA: I have told my husband that he is not the only one who can miss the signs of a heart attack. I was reading in my health magazine how women can be at risk and can leave their symptoms for too long. With me, that third time, before I went to hospital, I *knew* that I was not well, but I couldn't bring myself to go back to the doctors and all that rigamarole again.

DR DORIAN: Recognizing the signs of heart disease is a bit more complicated in women than in men. Women more often have what we call "atypical symptoms," which means feeling unwell in a nonspecific way, as opposed to men, who more commonly have chest pain or heaviness that occurs on exertion and subsides with rest, so-called classic symptoms. As a result, and because heart disease is less common in women at a younger age (unfortunately, women "catch up" to men with respect to CAD incidence by the eighth decade of life), the diagnosis is more difficult in women.

Again, the most important warning sign is *persistence* of symptoms, especially if they are not relieved by rest or nitro pills or spray. [Nitroglycerine is a common heart medication used to quickly relieve chest discomfort. See Part Two.]

ANNA: Well, I certainly think that "shock" is a good name for what we go through.

DR BAKER: The shock does help to protect the patient during medical treatment. As long as the family can keep calm, the medical team can do the rest. As you must know, there is no need to make other decisions at that time. It's when you get home that you will have your hands full!

ANNA: My husband and I have learned to work together after going through all those "events," as you call them. We certainly had enough practice! The good thing, in the end, is that, as a couple, we seem to be getting close again, and this makes us stronger to deal with any event that comes our way.

CHAPTER 4

Aftermath

aftermath *1. consequences, esp. unpleasant, 2. new grass growing after mowing*

—Oxford Dictionary of Current English

I wake to sleep, and take my waking slow.
I learn by going where I have to go.

—Theodore Roethke

Rose is lost

Rose was confused. She just wasn't sure what to do next. Her children, and her boss of forty-three years, were encouraging her to be more active, but she wasn't doing much of anything. It wasn't that she was upset; she just didn't feel well enough to do any of the things people were advising her to do, even cooking or visiting friends. After her heart attack and cardiac arrest at the shopping mall, she had spent a couple of weeks in the hospital. The physicians said that they were satisfied with her recovery, that she could go home, but would have "to take it easy." That was an understatement! Now, with her daughter living with her, Rose wondered whether, in fact, she could ever return to the secure life she had led before.

Meet Rose, a person who has had a major cardiac event that may have lasting effects on the way she conducts her life. As her story unfolds over the course of her journey, we will see if a good "quality of life" can be restored, despite permanent effects on her heart and residual limitations to her level of functioning. In Rose's case, her attitude is going to be crucial in coming to terms with changes in her life. Many of you will be less affected than Rose as your medical status is less severe; however, Rose speaks to us in an inspiring way, on how she copes. Rose shows the emotional disorientation of the aftermath that occurs at this time, even though she is not a particularly "emotional" person. The significant others are, as usual, "major players"; during the aftermath, which is a brief period, the family should be aware of an extra involvement with the patient, an involvement that can either be of no help, or of much benefit, to the patient. We'll conclude with a forum discussion with Rose and her daughter of the issues they found especially pertinent during their experience of the aftermath.

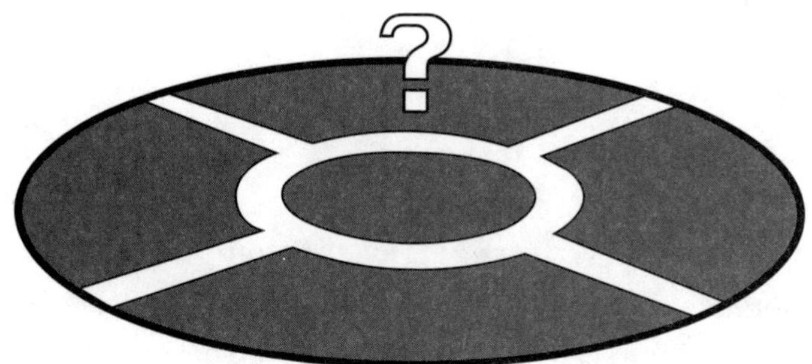

WHERE AM I?

DURING THE EVENT, so much is going on, and in such a relatively short space of time, that there is not much to *do*. Things are done *to* you. You are rendered safe in the context of nurses, doctors and what medical technology can offer to deal with any eventuality. For many who have suffered a cardiac event, there is precious little time between the initial relief of knowing you will be all right and the announcement that you will be leaving the sanctuary of physical safety. This period of relief is short-lived and is replaced with a feeling of bewilderment. For most, this is uncharted territory. Even those who have been down this road before have only the reassurance gathered from that one experience or series of experiences. Medically, your cardiac status has been stabilized, but you do not feel *well.* The family now awaits your arrival with expectancy and concern.

Homecoming is a return to a previous reality, but your own *sense* of reality has changed. As the shock wears off, the sense of *being lost* surfaces. For loved ones, this can be the most challenging time, as both feelings of fear and the need to protect the patient are paramount. This is a rather confusing time for patient and family, and we need to help you find your way out of this confusion and into a state of some clarity.

WHERE AM I MEDICALLY?

DURING THE INITIAL hospitalization phase, patients may not have the opportunity to have all of their questions answered. In acute-care hospitals, doctors are often very busy dealing with emergencies, or other patients in the first minutes or hours of a heart attack, and may have somewhat less time to spend with patients who are convalescing uneventfully. In large university-based teaching hospitals, patients may be cared for by a team of physicians in the coronary care unit and a different team in the ordinary hospital ward, thus coming into contact with very many doctors and nurses in rapid succession, and therefore may have great difficulty forming a bond with any one individual to whom they can turn with questions and concerns. Unfortunately, the hurly-burly of hospital activities is not well suited to quiet and thoughtful conversation between patients, their loved ones and their caregivers.

Don't be surprised if you're not sure what questions to ask, for in the first few days most patients concentrate on the present and the immediate future, and need to integrate the experience before they are able to consider the longer term. Remember, you will have many opportunities to ask questions after hospital discharge, when the real process of recuperation and rehabilitation begins. Following the initial acute phase of a heart attack or unstable angina, most patients' symptoms subside substantially or disappear completely, at least in the hospital. Patients begin to be up and about on the ward and they will be placed on a medication regimen similar to that they will receive as outpatients after discharge. However, the hospital is a protected environment with constant attention from doctors, nurses and other medical personnel. It is usually immediately before or after discharge that anxieties set in. This is especially true for patients who do not have a secure support system—family or friends—to help them manage in the early days after discharge. Many hospitals are able to arrange some form of care in the home, with visiting nurses or other individuals who can help the patient through this potentially difficult time.

By the time of hospital discharge, most patients will be completely free of chest discomfort. Occasionally there is some residual soreness, which is sometimes worse on deep breathing, caused by inflammation of the lining of the heart (known as *pericarditis*), which is unrelated to the arterial blockage itself. The bed rest, even though it may have lasted only a few days, and the effects of the event itself will often lead to generalized weakness, dizziness upon standing up, and some instability on walking. Expect that it will take you several days, or even a week or two, to "get your sea legs back," and especially that you will be lightheaded upon standing up suddenly. You also need to become adjusted to the routine of taking multiple medications upon your return home, and it is useful to develop a strategy to remember all your medications. Some patients find that taking them under exactly the same circumstances (for example, your morning pills before brushing your teeth, your evening pills at bedtime) is helpful; others use pillboxes with a time alarm, or other electrical gadgets your pharmacist can show you, which help remind you when to take your medications.

The time between your hospital discharge and your first scheduled visit with your cardiologist may be especially unsettling. Many patients have had an *exercise test* before hospital discharge, but generally this will be rather gentle and does not require rapid walking or jogging. You should be comfortable in knowing that you can perform everyday activities that take surprisingly little energy and pose relatively low stress to the heart. This includes taking out the garbage, walking around the house or up stairs, visiting friends, and indulging in sexual activity. We firmly believe that resumption of social and sexual activity is usually safe even relatively early after a heart event, although you will want to delay vigorous or sporting activities until after your first checkup and your more vigorous exercise test—usually six weeks after the event. Of course, your interest in sexual activity or socializing may be low after a heart attack, and you should not be surprised or feel guilty if you want to "retreat into your shell" at this time. However, if you are interested or feel up to it, it is not dangerous to resume these activities, and it may be worthwhile to encourage yourself to "get back to life," even if you're not sure you have the motivation, as it will help speed you toward recuperation.

At this time, although this is always true for patients with heart disease, you especially need to listen to your body without being overwhelmed by the signals that it gives you. For example, if you are extremely short of breath, feel like fainting or have severe chest discomfort, your body is clearly telling you to stop whatever you are doing and to seek medical attention. On the other hand, do not be surprised at minor aches and pains, at feeling generally without pep and down in the dumps—these discomforts will subside over the following weeks.

Remember that your family may not be used to dealing with a heart patient, and may be just as anxious as you are, if not more so, and inclined to be overprotective. Please be sure that your doctors speak to your loved ones about what is safe activity for you, so that you are not unnecessarily restricted because of their (understandable) fears.

WHERE AM I EMOTIONALLY?

IN THE MOVIE *Raising Arizona*, there is a scene in which a couple is attempting to escape through a tunnel, with a baby in hand. They are under the threat of capture. All of a sudden, the couple emerges into the sharp daylight of a humdrum town scene. Are they safe? The visual and emotional contrast of them being under threat in this "dark place," followed by a sudden return to an apparently safe and normal situation, is simultaneously jarring and exciting—a *disorienting* experience.

This early stage in the journey of recovery is characterized by *discordance*. Discordance can literally mean a clash of sounds or lack of harmony, which aptly describes an experience that results from a number of different feelings at the same time. Let us start with our physical feelings. You are familiar with how you regularly feel in your body. Now, things have changed; there will be sensations and symptoms that you are not used to having. The body has not yet returned to a stable state. It is unsettled. This is caused by the event itself, by the enforced inactivity in the hospital and immediately after, and by the medications that can subtly alter your internal thermometer. We all constantly receive signals from our body, which is "background" and doesn't command much attention from us. For example, we are all aware, if we concentrate on it, of our breathing, and even our heartbeat. Some of these sensations are briefly unpleasant, but we are not concerned about them if we are otherwise healthy. Patients who have recently been ill pay closer attention to the signals they pick up from their bodies, and often are unsure if these everyday sensations are normal or indicate recurrence of their illness.

As you try to deal with what is a new physical state for you, you are unsure about the implications of your sensations and symptoms, particularly if symptoms, such as chest pain, fatigue, shortness of breath or palpitations, keep recurring. So, there is caution and an associated wariness. You ask, what does this new state *mean*? There is the realization that not only has your body changed, but *you* have changed.

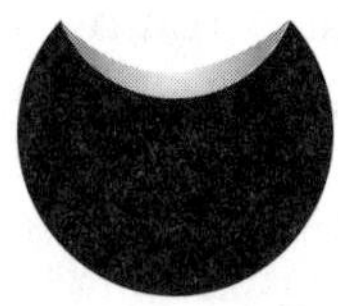

Fig. 4.1
Emotional Limbo —
Disorientation

Figure 4.1 illustrates what you go through emotionally during the aftermath. Again you see the circle that represents your emotional experience. However, here the area of protection that was prominent at the time of the event has started to recede. This has left some "raw" areas exposed, while other areas remain covered by an ever-diminishing protective film. This demonstrates the transitional phase of the aftermath and accounts for the sense of being emotionally disoriented at this time, a period that can usually be measured in days. Indeed, the aftermath is an in-between state, but is distinctive enough to warrant discussion as a separate phase.

But, just a minute, who am I? And what is going on? Where am I now? These existential questions sound dramatic but are a result of the underlying emotional state. It is one of confusion. Not one of *actual* confusion—you know the literal answers to these questions: "I am Joe Blow, I have just got home after a heart attack and I am starting to recover from it." So physically you are oriented, but emotionally you are not—you are betwixt and between. Your new way of living or coping in the world has not yet been established. For the moment, it is helpful to simply know that you are *in this phase*. You have just emerged from the tunnel, as it were; the sunlight is strong, life seems to be going on in a normal way for the rest of the world. Within days to weeks, what you have to deal with will become clearer. Now you must emotionally tide yourself through this brief period, follow your doctor's instructions and before you know it, you will be dealing with the challenges of the next phase (see Chapter 5).

FAMILY CONCERNS

FOR THE FAMILY, the aftermath is a very active phase. If you (as spouse) ever wanted to be chief cook and bottle washer, now is the time! But, in addition to all these roles, you yourself are going through your *own* journey. In the hospital you are included in the instructions and education about heart disease. You want to understand what is being told to your loved one, all that will impinge on your role as caregiver, as there will be a mantle of responsibility when the patient comes home. Your help can be invaluable if the patient does not comprehend everything that is told to him or her, as is often the case in the early stages when many are in an emotional state they describe as "dazed and confused." But you yourself may already be reacting to the cardiac event, a reaction that you may understand better when you become familiar with the next phase the patient will go through (see discussion of emotional response of recuperation in Chapter 5). To avoid repeating ourselves, we will only highlight one fairly typical scenario with cardiac patients.

On arrival home, the patient returns to a familiar environment—the usual people, the usual place. However, physically and emotionally, they do not feel the same as before. Like it or not, there will be a period of uncertainty. Is everything going to be okay? During this time, the spouse's concern is translated into a type of *watchfulness*, of scrutiny, where there is the understandable need to check on the patient. Initially, this is adaptive—meaning it is normal, even important, that this be done. However, if fear should override this attitude, then overprotectiveness can result, which is not healthy for the patient or spouse. This state has been termed "hypervigilance" and is classically seen in the aftermath. Sometimes it can be so extreme that the spouse won't let the patient go anywhere alone. This rapidly leads to the patient feeling "suffocated" and cannot continue for long without harm to the patient, the caregiver and their relationship; fortunately, this pattern tends to subside in almost all cases. We must accept that if the patient has been medically permitted to leave the safety of the hospital, then constant observation is not required. For this phase, though, it is normal, appropriate and helpful for the caregiver to generally observe and monitor the patient and to take what actions seem appropriate.

So, there is a natural caring that can spill over into protectiveness in the very early homecoming period. The spouse is the "parent"; the patient, the dependent "child" in the sense of showing dependent needs. This is a *temporary* situation, something that will need to change as the patient moves into the next phase, and toward independence.

Remember, the aftermath is a time when the patient feels unsafe, and their loved ones may feel unsafe about them. But awareness of this period of vulnerability will help to prepare the patient for the journey ahead.

FORUM (ROSE): Lost and found

In this forum, we examine the aftermath from the perspective of someone who lives alone and whose event had a substantial impact, but who experiences this phase in ways with which most can identify. Our theme here is the simple but important one of acknowledging the sense of being "lost," as this can start the process of finding the way on the journey to recovery.

Rose is a sixty-seven-year-old secretary who has worked for the same company for forty-three years. She continued to work full-time despite having angina, which she adjusted to well. She was shopping at a local mall, when she suddenly felt severe chest pain. Paramedics were summoned, and, just after they got there, she had a cardiac arrest from which she was shocked back to normal with *defibrillation.* In the hospital, she was told that she had had a large heart attack and had suffered substantial heart damage. Later, an *angiogram* showed that *bypass surgery* or *angioplasty* was not indicated, and although she was unlikely to suffer another heart attack, she would be left with significant heart damage. She was placed on several heart medications, and discharged after two weeks. She was told that, in time, she could still be eligible for a modified exercise program. Rose is very close to her three daughters, one of whom resides out of town. When Rose came home, her two daughters who live nearby alternated staying with her. Her oldest daughter accompanied Rose in this forum.

DAUGHTER: I am pleased you asked us to discuss this specific period, which you called "the Aftermath," as this was something that impacted on us quite a lot. Mom was really not herself and she needed someone there with her all the time. Do you remember what it was like, Mom?

ROSE: Well, I haven't lost my memory completely! Of course I do. I wasn't sure what was going to happen. I didn't feel myself, but I wasn't used to all that fuss and attention.

DR DORIAN: What was it like for the family at this time?

DAUGHTER: Frankly, it wasn't easy when Mom was in the hospital; but at least she was being well looked after by the medical staff. The problems started when she came home and we weren't sure how well she was going to get. I was most interested in what you described as a quite typical reaction from family members, in that we became very protective toward Mom. For a few days, I wouldn't let Mom out of my sight.

ROSE: Yes, I found that a bit irritating, but at the same time I was relieved that you were looking after me.

DR BAKER: It sounds like it *was* necessary to closely monitor your mother's progress, especially in those days just after returning home, given her heart condition. We expect, at least initially, for there to be *some* scrutiny of the patient, but this contrasts with the type of pattern we described where this can become smothering.

DAUGHTER: No, I don't think it was to that extent. Besides, once Mom got over the insecurity of not knowing whether she would be okay, and especially whether she could carry on living in the house on her own, she didn't need us very much. But it's true what you say—there is a big question mark about those early days, when you are not sure what's going to happen.

DR DORIAN: Rose, did you feel confused, as we described in the chapter?

ROSE: Well, I'm not someone to dwell on things, you know. I guess I was confused with not knowing about the future. Those were difficult days because I wasn't sure if I could live on my own again.

DR BAKER: I can hear that your independence is important to you.

ROSE: It's everything to me. I knew it was best to have a companion for a little while, but, as my daughter will tell you, I prefer to look after others—not have them look after me!

DAUGHTER: I wouldn't contradict that, Mom!

DR BAKER: This is a challenging time for both patient and family. The patient leaves the safety of the hospital environment and there is insecurity all around. At the same time, responsibility is felt by the caregivers.

DAUGHTER: That's for sure. I don't know if Mom cares to recall the second night when she came home. My fourteen-year-old was giving us a hard time and I just had to go home to calm things down.

ROSE: I wasn't sure if you'd ever bring up that evening.

DAUGHTER: It's always been "Don't worry about me" with my mom, so this time I took her at her word, but secretly I felt uneasy. Then, when I got to my home, I was distracted by teenage tantrums.

ROSE: You know, I never told you, but *that* night was a long one. I was feeling very tired and weak, and I naturally wasn't my perky self—in fact, I felt a bit strange. So I turned on the television to my favorite soap, but I couldn't concentrate. I just knew I wasn't going to call my daughters, so then I remembered my neighbor Ida. I gave her a call and she also couldn't leave the apartment, but she talked to me for an hour on the telephone. Then I felt better, and so I fell asleep on the sofa and awoke just as you came back.

DAUGHTER: That's why you were there! I had thought—Just like Mom! She's just had a heart attack and she's waiting up for me!

DR BAKER: It's good that, for most, the aftermath lasts only for a brief period of time, when we are always reminding patients and their families to "hang on to their hats."

DR DORIAN: Coming home from a hospital, especially after a large heart attack, can be disconcerting. Most patients feel quite shaky, and it takes some time getting used to their new situation of requiring a fair amount of medication, having less energy than they are used to, and coming to terms with their disabilities. Importantly, there is almost always improvement from the time of hospital discharge until two or four weeks later, especially these days, when patients are discharged from the hospital soon after their initial attack. This disorientation is often more profound in patients who have had complications, such as a cardiac arrest. Fortunately, a cardiac arrest in the throes of a heart attack does not imply a poor future outcome, but it does make the initial adjustment more difficult.

ROSE: Well, I am pleased that you mentioned that. Not only for me, mind you, but for anyone who might read this after going through what I did, as I think I did quite well by the end of the "journey," as you put it.

DAUGHTER: My mother has a way of accepting things and not focusing on what she has had to give up. She had been quite a dynamo before this all happened.

ROSE: Well, what's the point of dwelling on the past? I think it always best to look at the glass half full, not half empty. Besides, I see it as three-quarters full!

DR BAKER: Rose, you do show how a positive attitude can improve recovery. Do you want a last word on that time, after the doctors said you were out of danger and then when you came home?

ROSE: I did feel strange *and* insecure, *and* I am glad it's over with!

CHAPTER 5

Recuperation

recuperate: *1. recover from illness, exhaustion, loss 2. regain [health, a loss]*

—OXFORD DICTIONARY OF CURRENT ENGLISH

What wound did ever heal but by degrees?

—OTHELLO

Is Mary healing?

"Let's get on with it!" she thought. "There's always so much going on in my life; another thing should be no problem!" Mary did not linger too long with the fact that that "thing" was a heart attack. She was an executive, with a hundred-and-one commitments, deadlines and more deadlines, a couple of teenagers and a new love in her life—her boyfriend of the past six months.

Three weeks ago, Mary had suddenly been forced to deal with a part of her life that was never before a concern—her health. Her heart attack came out of the blue, just as she was preparing for a business trip; at the time, it was a bit of a shock, but soon what had happened was receding in her mind as she filled it with preoccupations about work. She was eager to get going with the new rehab program.

Naturally, she wanted to see more of her boyfriend; momentarily she wondered if he would leave her. A week later, Mary was unhappy. She realized she was much slowed down.

Mary will confront "the high road and the low road" of recuperation. Although hers may typify the experience of many, Mary's version of this phase is uniquely hers. If you see yourself in Mary's story, you are someone who doesn't like to reflect too much on what is going on—"a person of action." We will find out, though, that without pacing yourself, you can "hit a wall." You will also learn that, if you cannot solve problems as you want them to be solved, as quickly as you would like, you will get frustrated, and possibly irritated or even angry, if that is your bent.

Mary is also recognizable to so many of us whose family setup is not "Mom, Dad, the three kids, the dog and the white picket fence." In modern society, "the family" is characterized by variations and permutations that can be the "joker in the pack" when a cardiac event intrudes into our lives.

Finally, we will see whether Mary will achieve one of the goals of recuperation—the notion of "balance," which applies to physical state, emotional experience and relations with loved ones and work environment.

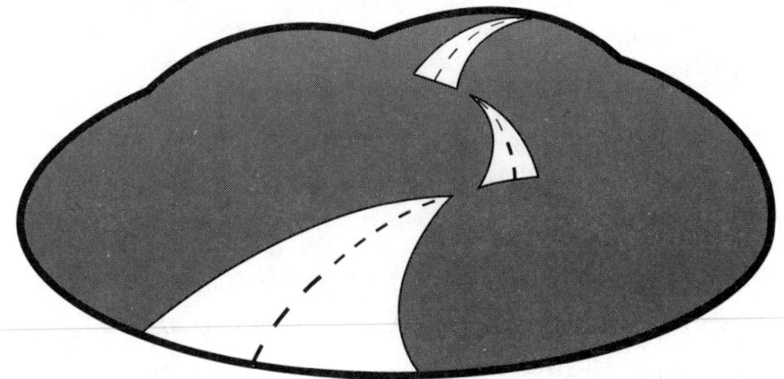

The bumpy road

We now move on to one of the two main themes in the journey of recovery after a cardiac event—recuperation, which refers to a period of *healing*. This phase is not clearly distinguishable from the others, but it is useful to identify for those who are on this journey. As we show, there is some contrast between the way the body heals and the way the mind reacts. While the body heals in a fairly consistent way, during this phase the mind goes through what is often the most challenging time—that of "reaction." The most prominent emotional experiences include *normal fear* or anxiety; *sadness* in response to what many perceive as a loss; low mood or *depression*; and *anger*, a familiar response that unfortunately has been neglected in the context of recovering from a cardiac event. While much will depend on the progress of the patient, in general the caregivers will heal more quickly than the patient. It is important for the family to be aware of the particular hazards of this phase for the patient, a phase whose main aim will be "achieving a balance" of both physical and emotional symptoms, and a sense of coherence both in the patient and in the family system. (We further discuss the emotional and cardiac aspects of healing in "Heart to Mind" in Part Two.) We'll conclude this chapter with a forum that highlights how healing can be a bumpy ride and how balance can be restored.

THE BODY HEALS

FORTUNATELY, HEART MUSCLE heals quite quickly—in about two to three weeks. After the healing is complete, the heart attack is physically "over and done with," and the heart's future depends on the risk of undergoing another event. Although patients quite naturally tend to dwell on the remote and recent past, it is appropriate at this time to concentrate on the future, including recuperation and rehabilitation. Both allow the possibility of a healthier and potentially happier life even though the heart is not as physically strong as it once was.

Many patients are not sure how quickly they can return to their previous activities, and what they are "allowed to do." The best and simplest advice is: "Listen to your body." For the majority of individuals, there is little danger in everyday physical activities even shortly after a heart attack, provided that they do not cause undue shortness of breath, dizziness, chest discomfort or palpitations. Most patients are quite capable of looking after themselves; can be up and about in the house, including climbing stairs; and can even go out for short gentle walks or visits. Provided there are no complications, most patients can return to their previous activities in four to six weeks.

Naturally, since heart damage invariably occurs with a heart attack, the ability to be physically active may be restricted after the event, sometimes permanently. The extent of actual limitation will vary from person to person, but is rarely extreme. Most patients will undergo some form of *exercise testing* at four to six weeks following a heart attack, and their ability to exercise under supervision will allow the cardiologist or the rehabilitation clinic personnel to offer an "exercise prescription." Most patients are pleasantly surprised that they can walk briskly without significant symptoms, even at one month.

For patients who have had *unstable angina*, more intensive testing is common, and procedures are often performed either during the initial hospitalization or in the days to weeks following discharge. Since, in some senses, unstable angina is "a heart attack waiting to happen," the location, extent and severity of narrowing of the heart arteries often need to be precisely measured with a *coronary angiogram* (for details on this and other procedures, see Part Two). This very important test allows the doctor to precisely identify the location and appearance of the narrowings that are present, and is very helpful, even necessary, in guiding future therapy. In general, there are three possible outcomes of the angiogram.

The type and severity of the narrowings may be such that *coronary artery bypass surgery* is advised. This decision also takes into account whether the patient's symptoms have continued despite medical treatment. In this surgical procedure, the narrowed segments of the major arteries are *bypassed* (i.e., a detour is made around these narrowings or blockages) using veins from the legs, which can be safely removed, or arteries usually taken from the inside of the chest wall. This surgery has a high probability of success and a relatively low chance of serious complications. It is, however, major surgery and will be associated with some anxiety during the waiting period and discomfort in the recuperation phase, and requires psychological adjustment after the surgery. The overall results of this surgery are excellent, and most patients no longer have chest pains or discomforts, and are at low risk of serious heart events in the months to years following successful bypass.

In many patients, the narrowings of the arteries are such that the artery can be opened up from the *inside*, using a procedure known as *percutaneous transluminal coronary angioplasty (PTCA)*. This is sometimes known as the "balloon procedure" and is performed by sliding a small, flexible soft wire through the large arteries from the leg through to the heart, and passing this wire through the area of narrowing. A tube with a deflated balloon is then threaded over this wire, and the balloon positioned so that it is sitting "inside the blockage." The balloon is then inflated at pressure, "opening up" the area formerly narrowed. The procedure is usually successful, although not every patient is a candidate due to technical limitations such as extremely long narrowings, narrowings in blood vessels inaccessible to the wire or balloon, or narrowings in arteries too small for the balloon to fit through. Recent developments have improved the long-term success of this procedure. Formerly, a fair number of patients experienced *restenosis*, a reoccurrence of the original narrowing, in the months following the procedure. The risk of this can be reduced by using *coronary stents*, a type of wire mesh "scaffolding" which is introduced into the artery at the previous site of blockage, and expands to "hold the artery open," allowing better blood flow and reducing the chance of renewed blockage. Also, intravenous medications are now available that can be used in some cases to reduce the risk of renewed *occlusion* or blockage.

Often, neither bypass surgery nor angioplasty is suggested. This need not be a cause for despair. In many cases, a blocked artery spontaneously reopens after a heart attack, and there is no need for bypassing or opening up this artery afterwards. In some cases, the body performs its own "natural bypasses," known as *collaterals*, which take blood from an adjacent normal artery to portions of heart muscle normally supplied by an artery that is now blocked. In some cases, only a small artery is blocked and the remaining arteries function normally, and there is little risk of future events. In all these situations, bypass surgery or angioplasty would be of no value, and is not required, but the outcome is still very good. Occasionally, however, the heart damage and the type and location of blockages are such that neither bypass surgery nor angioplasty can be safely or effectively performed. The outlook is not necessarily poor for even these patients; although medications can usually not reverse blockages, they can stabilize the condition for months, or even years, allowing patients to resume satisfying and productive lives.

In almost all instances, cardiac medications will be prescribed—after these procedures, or instead of them. These drugs, and the importance of taking them, are described below and in Part Two.

The way patients feel and their *prognosis* (their medical future) are related to the consequences of having had a heart attack or unstable angina. In general terms, patients can experience three types of problems. First, there are problems of "plumbing." These relate to the consequences of having narrowed or blocked coronary arteries, which, in turn, may lead to *angina pectoris* (chest pain caused by lack of oxygen to the heart), or shortness of breath, which may culminate in another heart attack, or another attack of unstable angina. The likelihood of such problems depends on the state of the arteries after the initial event, and the success of the subsequent treatment.

A second concern is that of the extent of scarring in the heart, usually measured in terms of the *left ventricular function* (the strength of the pumping ability of the heart). The more extensive the scarring, in general the less the ability to exercise, and the more fatigue and breathlessness that will follow exercise. However, as pointed out below, even patients with extensive scarring can benefit from some degree of activity, if done with supervision. Very severe weakness of the heart muscle can lead to *congestive heart failure*, a condition characterized by shortness of breath, sometimes severe and at rest, nighttime cough or inability to lie flat, ankle swelling and extreme fatigue. This condition, sometimes associated with "water in the lungs," usually needs urgent therapy, but with treatment many patients can expect to regain the level of health they had prior to developing the condition.

The third type of problem encountered by patients after a heart attack is changes in heart rhythms, known as *arrhythmias*, considered to be electrical disturbances of heart function. Most commonly these are manifested as *premature ventricular contractions* (extra beats), which are usually not perceived by the patient but may indicate a risk for more serious rhythm disturbances. Occasionally, patients may have a "short circuit," known as *ventricular tachycardia*, which can cause very rapid palpitations, lightheadedness, and even loss of consciousness. Fortunately, these serious rhythm disturbances are rare. However, any episode of marked dizziness and near fainting or complete loss of consciousness should be reported to your doctor immediately.

Somewhat confusingly, there are many medications that are known to be beneficial after a heart attack. Patients often must take several kinds of pills, at various times of day, and might not understand why they were prescribed. Some of these medications may in fact cause minor side effects, at least early on, and patients may wonder if they would not be better off not taking them. Some of them do not make patients feel better in the short run, even though they are protective in the long run. It is thus important to understand the purpose of heart medications prescribed for you, and their ultimate benefit.

Aspirin should be taken by almost all patients following a heart attack or unstable angina, unless they have allergies or experience severe stomach upset after taking ASA. This drug prevents blood elements known as *platelets* from sticking together in clumps and causing clot formation and arterial blockage. ASA reduces the incidence of heart attack and death in patients with unstable angina and other cardiac events. Another group of drugs that are undoubtedly effective are *beta blockers*, drugs that counteract the actions of adrenaline on the heart and the rest of the body. They reduce the risk of future heart attacks and death, probably because adrenaline, a "fight or flight" or "stress" hormone, is damaging to the heart's circulatory function and to the heart muscle itself. The complex defense mechanism that the body employs to combat physical stress includes manufacturing large quantities of stress hormones such as adrenaline that cause blood vessels to constrict, the heart to pump faster and harder, and the blood elements to be stickier and more liable to clot. This response of course protects us from the danger of bleeding to death, for example, when injured, as must have been the case when our ancestors were hunter-gatherers.

However, these days, most of us hunt bargains at the mall or gather doughnuts in the bakery section of the supermarket.

After a heart attack, the concentrations of these stress hormones in the blood increase, but the stress is not acute (as is the case after an injury), but chronic and ongoing, owing to heart muscle weakness. As a result, the production of adrenaline and other stress hormones, which are known to be toxic to the heart over time, continues. Thus beta blockers, which slow the heart rate and, in fact, weaken the heart muscle pump in the short term, are protective in the long term by putting the heart to rest, so to speak. We know that the slower the heart rate, that is, the fewer beats per minute, the longer patients seem to live after a heart attack. The adage that one has only a certain number of heartbeats in a lifetime and one can use them up slowly or quickly may be not far from the truth. Getting angry or upset, for example, increases the heart rate and should be avoided for this reason, among others. Although exercise increases the heart rate temporarily, individuals who exercise regularly generally have lower heart rates than those who do not, even though for brief periods *during* exercise their heart rates are higher. Thus, unless there are specific reasons against it, the vast majority of patients who have had a heart attack should remain on beta blockers, probably indefinitely.

Patients who have had a moderately large or large heart attack may also be prescribed a category of drugs known as *ACE inhibitors*, drugs that indirectly counteract the action of another substance known as *angiotensin*, which is a powerful constrictor of blood vessels and which is also a "stress hormone" and raises blood pressure. Since blood pressure may also be elevated after a heart attack, patients benefit from medications that lower it.

The issue of *cholesterol* is relatively complex. Recent scientific studies have suggested that even normal levels of cholesterol (i.e., normal for the average North American) may be too high for someone who has coronary artery disease. Levels previously thought to be "average" are seen as undesirably high in those who have had a heart attack, and the levels of cholesterol that are now set as a target are in fact low compared with population norms. Thus many doctors believe that almost all patients who have experienced a CAD event should be on some cholesterol-lowering drug, unless their cholesterol is extremely low to begin with. Avoiding dietary fats and dietary cholesterol can lower the blood cholesterol to some degree, but probably not enough to achieve this end.

Many patients may be prescribed a group of drugs known as *calcium channel blockers*, drugs that relax the blood vessel wall and lower blood pressure, and decrease the stress on the heart. These drugs can be quite effective in combating angina, but have not clearly been shown to prolong life. Similarly, nitroglycerin or its derivatives are very effective at reducing angina, but may not prolong life. The most commonly used drug for angina is nitroglycerin given under the tongue by tablet or as a mouth spray, and it works almost immediately to relieve chest discomfort caused by lack of blood and oxygen to the heart (angina) and can be used as often as necessary if chest discomfort or pain keeps recurring. Some other patients may receive drugs to prevent heart rhythm disturbances, known as *antiarrhythmic drugs*. These are drugs used to prevent excessively rapid or irregular heartbeats.

Sexual and other activities

Most patients and their spouses, albeit in their different ways, are concerned about when and how to resume the activities of daily living, whether routine or vigorous, and especially sexual activity.

It is of course impossible to give advice that applies to all patients, but some general notions are useful to all. Daily activities such as showering, dressing, walking about the house (including up and down one or two flights of stairs) and cooking require relatively little effort, and are rarely risky or difficult for heart patients. Even at one week after a heart attack, most patients are well enough to go home and carry out activities of daily living, including mildly strenuous activities such as vacuuming, unloading groceries and doing other housework.

Although sexual activity is considered by many to be strenuous, the actual workload or stress on the heart is similar to that experienced during a brisk walk and poses little danger to the vast majority of patients, even soon after a heart attack. Sexual activity *is* intense (as opposed to strenuous) and can lead to symptoms such as shortness of breath, palpitations or chest pain. As for any other activity, let your body be the guide. If you experience symptoms, slow your activity and consult your doctor.

A digression about sex and heart disease is important here. Recent research shows that men (there is unfortunately no comparable information available for women, but the information very likely applies equally) who engage in regular sexual activity (two times per week for those of you who are counting) live longer than men who do not. Our interpretation is that sexual activity is just one way of expressing or receiving intimacy, and it is the intimate, hopefully loving and committed, relationship with your partner that supports and protects your heart. It is important to remember that there are many ways to show affection, and that sexual intercourse is just one of these ways; physical closeness, hugging or even holding hands can be a great source of comfort to patients with heart events and, in this sense, we strongly encourage physical contact between our patients and their loved ones.

Impotence (inability to achieve or maintain an erection) is common among men with heart disease, especially after a heart attack. Neither partner should expect the same sexual performance and intensity as before the illness, at least not in the early days. As for all other symptoms or concerns, do not hesitate to discuss this with your doctor to obtain advice that applies specifically to you.

THE MIND REACTS

WHEN YOU ARE given a local anesthetic (say, when you are to receive stitches for a deep cut), it is effective during the procedure, but you may notice that, as it wears off, an inverse effect occurs: the area becomes *more* sensitive than it was before. While the event is going on, there is protection, but once the protective layering is removed, a *release* occurs. It pays to be aware of this recoil mechanism; otherwise, it can hit you in the face! Figure 5.1 shows that the cover formed by the impact of the event (see "numbing" in Figure 3.3, page 29) is now removed, and that the person is now emotionally "exposed to the elements." As a result, there is a *delayed response* to the event that took place some days ago. The response will vary greatly, depending on the particular event and individual concerned. Given this large variation in what we can expect, the general term "reaction" is used to describe this emotional response that usually takes weeks to months to complete. For a number of patients, some remnants of it can persist into the next phase of the journey (see Chapter 6).

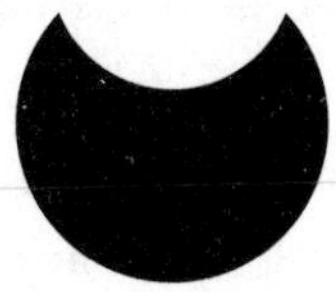

Fig. 5.1
Exposed to the elements

We can see that as the body starts to heal, the mind may, in contrast, start to react. This discrepancy between the timing of the healing of the body and of the mind is not uncommon, but it is necessary to be aware of it—particularly the strange things the mind can get up to—and to be aware that you may *overreact*, which can have a negative effect in your situation. In other words, you may read too much into what may be normal for this phase. Labeling an experience as "normal" does not mean that one can simply dismiss it, and we encourage you to find out more about the common emotional reactions that take place during this time. There are states of mind, and here we refer particularly to clinical depression, to which one needs to be alerted, and we will highlight them in this chapter and in Part Two. For the family, recuperation is an adjustment period that can proceed smoothly or not, depending on the makeup of the significant others, the patient and, of course, the circumstances. Flexibility is going to be an invaluable asset for the loving family member, but this is not always realistic or possible. This is a vulnerable time, but with medical evaluation and treatment, it will pass.

Fear

Fear is a normal response to threat. We feel afraid if something is threatening us. We have all experienced fear before and in the case of heart disease and especially during a cardiac event, it would be unusual not to be fearful. Perhaps anxiety is a more appropriate term. The experience is the same—a nervous, scared and shaky feeling. It affects the thinking in the form of worry and poor concentration, and it manifests in the body as muscle tension or chest pain, palpitations, stomach nerves and sweating (see Anxiety, Part Two).

Fear is often understood in terms of its time reference. In our "normal" lives we live in the present, but are influenced by the past and the future. For example, we are affected by the meal we have just had or, say, an argument that has bothered us. We are also influenced by what has been happening recently, such as pressure at work; a troubled or happy marriage; and, on a deeper level, by the more distant past, in terms of our personal history, or what has helped to make us who we are today. In a related way, we are also affected by the future. We look forward to a meeting with our loved ones or we may dread an encounter with someone we see as our nemesis. We think of what we may do this evening or next weekend, or eagerly anticipate a forthcoming trip. But despite all these influences, we are genuinely rooted to what is going on *now*.

For some time after the event, a patient's *sense* of time becomes disturbed. Patients are much affected, and may be shaken by what has taken place ("shaken" is particularly apt because fear characteristically involves a shaky feeling). But, even more importantly, they wonder whether it *will happen again*. So, the past (the cardiac event), and especially the future (anticipating another event), impinge on one's consciousness and take away some of the normality of being in the here-and-*now* that we take for granted at other times. But you need not be alarmed; your perception of time will normalize as you proceed on your journey of recovery.

Anxiety itself can give rise to the *same* symptoms that we see after a cardiac event—chest pain; shortness of breath; lack of concentration; and a cold, clammy feeling. As anxiety is often the response to a threat, if physical symptoms (perceived as threatening) occur, then anxiety will occur. Thus, a "vicious circle" of anxiety and physical symptoms triggering each other can be set in motion. We need to avoid this potential spiral by recognizing and dealing with it when it occurs. (See "Heart to Mind," page 246, and in Part Two, page 206.)

Sadness

In the wake of a cardiac event, all patients go through a time of contemplation, when they start to process what has been lost. Despite how it feels at the time, many of these losses are *perceived* and not real. Sadness is the normal response to loss—and we can expect *some* sadness; however, it doesn't have to linger long. The trouble is that we don't know at the time how things will turn out. Many will unintentionally exaggerate their losses; some will shut them out. But one loss is a genuine one—the loss of the sense of being "invulnerable" that we often carry around with us. Now that that bubble has been burst by the cardiac event, patients feel that things will "never be the same." In one sense, this is correct, as awareness of being a heart patient is permanent. New or recurrent heart disease can injure the "sense of self" that patients previously had. The illness tears at the fabric of the self, and most realize that, although the fabric can be mended, it can never be *exactly* the same again. Thus, the challenge of recuperation is to feel "whole" again. Successful recovery is centered on the search for a new, and perhaps better, equilibrium, once the initial shock has subsided. The knowledge that so many others have CAD, that people are living long lives and that these lives are usually of a good quality, is very heartening, if you'll excuse the pun.

So we ask ourselves, what are the losses over which we feel such sadness? Losses are perceived whenever there is a change in the role for the protagonist (you) as spouse, provider, lover, friend, parent, child or in any other capacity. During the emotional reaction of recuperation, there is an exaggerated sense that "all is lost" or "nothing is going to be as it was." While the loss of the old identity is real, much of what saddens you is *perceived* loss and you should adjust to it in time. The word "grief" can be used, in the sense that something is missed that seems irretrievable. Many patients referred to us over a decade ago thought they were "done for." They might have been told that they were not candidates for surgical intervention or they perhaps had had repeated cardiac arrests. We still see these patients on occasion, which shows that their original fears were unfounded. Their days were not numbered, but some losses are inevitable.

Sadness, being a normal response, will subside over time. However, a different state, intertwined with sadness, may need further attention—*low* or *depressed mood.*

Low mood

At times, the distinction between sadness and low mood is blurred; both can be present simultaneously. Your mood goes down when you have the feeling that the world is "on top" of *you*, rather than the reverse. Instead of being "on top of the world," you think you have lost control of your life. This feeling of not being capable, of incapacity, is linked with low mood or unhappiness. In the early stages of the recovery from a cardiac event like heart attack, this feeling is common and can be quite normal. When your ability to engage in normal activities or work seems threatened, it is not surprising that you feel frustration and unhappiness.

How bad does it get? How long does the low mood go on? These are questions we always ask, as for the CAD patient it seems that some forms of depression are linked to cardiac outcome. The problem is sorting out what is a "normal" depression, about which one can be reassured, and what is more serious depression, which will need specific treatment.

The main qualifiers in assessing depression are *severity* and *persistence*. Some people seem to have an unhappiness that is not severe but appears to go on and on, a condition we call *persistent low mood.* We don't fully understand this, but it may be related to mood states that occurred prior to the cardiac event. More commonly patients experience normal periods of sadness relating to what has happened to them, and low mood relating to feelings of incapacity. Over time, these feelings will subside; flare-ups, though, are to be expected. As you will see, depression and fatigue is a pattern that is now being better recognized (see below, and "Heart to Mind" in Part Two).

Joe is stalled (Clinical depression)

Joe just couldn't see the bright side. The future seemed bleak; he criticized himself for weakness. Later, during moments of clarity, he realized that this was unfair, but for the most part he just couldn't help himself. His main problem, though, was that after his heart attack he found it hard to get himself going. That situation dragged on for weeks. He had little interest and pleasure in things, things he usually loved to do, and his thinking was slow—like "a snail with a broken leg," someone had noted. He was being "carried" at work; his partners didn't complain about this, but Joe was sure that at some point they would just get fed up with him and remove him from the partnership.

Joe, one of the Select Six, happens to represent one out of six of all of those who have had a heart attack. (The prevalence of such symptoms may be different for those who have had cardiac events other than heart attack.) Joe still does not know it, but he has a *clinical depression.* That means he has a constellation of symptoms centered around depressed mood and low interest. The symptoms may vary, but a certain number of them must be present for the depression to be classified as "clinical" and therefore requiring treatment. The good news is, clinical depression is eminently treatable!

We discuss clinical depression in more detail in Part Two, but we do not expect patients to diagnose themselves. If symptoms of depression are severe or persistent, a consultation with a health professional is required. "Severe" means feeling so bad that you cannot cope, sometimes to the extent that you feel self-destructive in some way. "Persistent" conventionally means that symptoms have been present for two weeks, most of the day, nearly every day. Clinical depression tends to linger for months if not treated, is by definition linked to a very poor quality of life, and can get worse over time and compound the physical illness already present. Who needs this?! Research is starting to demonstrate that the one out of six patients after heart attack who develops a clinical depression is more likely to have a worse cardiac outcome than those who do not become clinically depressed. For patients who experienced other cardiac events, cardiac outcome is not as clearly associated with clinical depression. It is difficult to prove that treating depression will improve *cardiac* outcome and lessen the risk of further attacks, or even death, given that so many other factors significantly affect outcome, including heart functioning. One thing we do know: depression responds to interventions. For moderate to severe depression, antidepressants can be effective. Mild to moderate depression can respond well to a type of talking treatment (cognitive therapy) (see Part Two).

More doctors are starting to recognize clinical depression after a cardiac event, but unfortunately many patients have languished untreated for months on end. The diagnosis is quite simple, as is the choice of treatment. The decision to treat because of heart disease is not usually difficult, given the newer antidepressants and newer talking treatments. Before a patient is prescribed antidepressants, the cardiologist should be contacted and caution needs to be exercised with patients who have recently had a cardiac event, especially heart attack. Patients will need to be aware that side effects often occur in the early stages, but usually subside and are not usually severe enough to discontinue the medication. The response rate is 70 percent after about one month of treatment, as antidepressants take time to work. However, with persistence, there is invariably an acceptable result—usually a return to a completely normal emotional state, although it must be remembered that patients will still be responding to the effects of a cardiac event. Research is currently under way to examine the effects of a type of counseling (cognitive therapy) that appears promising for the depressed cardiac patient, especially those with milder depressions. In addition, researchers are examining modified versions of this treatment that can be combined with group approaches (see Part Two, specifically Depression, page 210, and Chapter 12, Joe, page 281).

In discussing low mood (see above), we referred to patients who have ongoing or *persistent* symptoms of mild depression. Even though this type of depression is milder than the clinical type, patients who experience it also seem to have their cardiac outcome affected, and so we are interested in treating these patients as well. It is likely that, for these patients especially, talking treatments will be the first choice, before antidepressants are considered. After heart attack, one out of six patients will have persistent low mood; so, altogether one-third of all such patients may need some form of treatment for depression. If you are experiencing a bout of low mood that will not go away, please read the discussion of depression in Part Two. Remember, response to treatment is usually excellent.

Anger

In the research on mind and heart, much has been written about the possible effects of ongoing anger and hostility as a "risk factor" for CAD. In other words, people who are constitutionally angry or hostile may be more susceptible to heart attack than those who are more even-tempered. This theory is still being investigated (see Chapter 6 and Part Two). However, many patients recuperating from a cardiac event report having angry feelings during the weeks *after* the event.

"Why me?" is the universal outcry. "Why not the guy next door, who has so many more risk factors, ignores his wife and is mean to his mother-in-law?!" What we hear from patients is an existential cry at the unfairness of what has been handed to them in their lives. This lament often surfaces within weeks of the cardiac event and is very responsive to a sympathetic ear. There is not much that the listener has to *do* initially, besides being prepared to listen, with empathy. However, the positive impact of having this anger acknowledged (or "validated") cannot be overstated, because a major blow to the sense of self has occurred and, in the early stages of reaction, many CAD patients feel their sense of self, their self-esteem, or the way they judge themselves, has been shaken. This won't last forever, but it can linger for weeks or months, until the next phase has taken good effect (see Chapter 6). For those in whom the anger *persists*, a different tack has to be taken. We address the question of anger management in general in Chapter 6 and, in a more focused way, in Part Two, but the point we wish to make here is that anger is a natural response to a cardiac event. If you can acknowledge it, and understand it, it will often subside on its own.

Anger continues for various reasons. Some people (maybe one out of five) are simply more aggressive than others. Associated with aggression is an underlying mistrust of others and a general cynicism about people and what one can expect out of life. When those who have this tendency experience a cardiac event—and particularly if stabilization of their medical state has, for some reason, been delayed, as was the case for Anna (see Chapter 3)—bitterness and anger, felt inwardly or expressed outwardly, can be expected. As we have seen, once the physical state has become stabilized, these attitudes and behaviors are likely to subside. As well, when such patients have committed to rehabilitation, these energies can be harnessed to more healthy ends. However, if the anger persists, there is ample evidence that patients would benefit from, both emotionally and in the long term in their cardiac outcome, instruction in the techniques of anger management (see Chapter 6 and Part Two).

FAMILY MATTERS

RECUPERATION CAN BE a bumpy ride for a patient's spouse, family and social and collegial network. The patient who is recuperating from a cardiac event is particularly changeable emotionally in terms of anxiety, sadness, low mood and anger. We have to remember that the mood of the significant other is changeable as well, but usually for a shorter time and less severely. But not all get off so lightly. There will be a stronger emotional response if the spouse or any family member is the "symptom bearer" on behalf of the patient. This means that it is not the patient but the family member who takes the brunt of being emotionally reactive in the family. Of course, much will depend on the actual physical state of the patient. Things go more smoothly if the patient is medically stable, or at least "stably unstable," which means that symptoms do occur but are recognizable and are deemed not serious by the physician. As well, a lot depends on the people involved—the patient and family members—and the relationships between them. Many relationships are not flexible enough; they function well when things go relatively smoothly, but a cardiac event can disturb the emotional equilibrium of a relationship. As we pointed out in

Chapter 4, "Aftermath," spouses can become overly involved with the patient's situation, which can be manifested as overconcern, or "hovering over" the patient ("hypervigilance"). This situation can be highly distressing to the patient, robbing him or her of privacy and independence as the spouse or other family members watch every step and limit every activity. Following the aftermath stage, this behavior pattern usually subsides, but in certain cases it can continue, to the detriment of both patient and caregiver. If both spouses are symptomatic or troubled, a potentially dangerous "spiral" can occur, with each person feeding off the negativity of the other and making things worse. Almost all patients will go through the bumpiness of emotional reaction. However, significant others may experience a rough ride as well, especially if acceptable reliance of the patient on the spouse at the start becomes unacceptable dependence, continuing into the weeks, and especially the months, following the cardiac event.

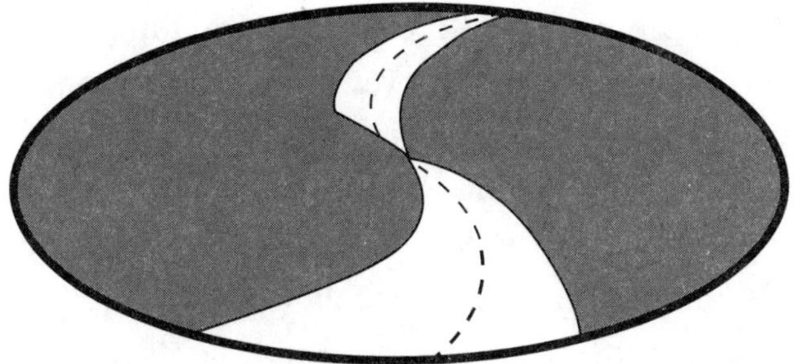

Road smoothing out

ACHIEVING A BALANCE

How do you know when you are getting better? The final word on your health must belong to your physicians, but we wish to raise a theme here that we have found helpful on the journey from event to recovery, especially in preparing for the next phase, rehabilitation.

An event disturbs the balance within the body, from which the body needs to recover. Symptoms such as chest pain, fatigue, shortness of breath and palpitations indicate to us that something is off-kilter. The actual journey back to health is taken with the guidance of your physicians, who can follow the great strides in the medical management of CAD to improve outcome; however, even when this has been achieved, it is not the end of the story. First, we have to get used to the new physical state; if symptoms are negligible, then, of course, it is much easier. Second, the feelings of fear, sadness, low mood and anger we have described as common manifestations of emotional reaction after a cardiac event can take time before settling down. Finally, within the family system, an upset has occurred that will take time to resolve.

So, in a theoretical sense, the challenge of recuperation is to restore a balance within the physical, emotional and family systems. This is not instantly achievable; efforts toward it must be sustained over time. There is considerable overlap between this phase and the next one, rehabilitation, especially in terms of starting physician-recommended activities. However, we have found that patients and their significant others appreciate knowing what they are going through in the weeks and months following a cardiac event. Furthermore, there comes a time when attitude becomes crucial in the recovery process. We are now approaching a junction point in the journey to recovery. Achieving balance is an important step toward this crossroad.

After the initial, uncertain, variable aftermath of a heart attack, during which the long-term treatment plans will have been made and carried out, patients face a period where they will need to gather their inner strength and head toward rehabilitation. It is at the end of this approximately four-to-eight-week period after the acute

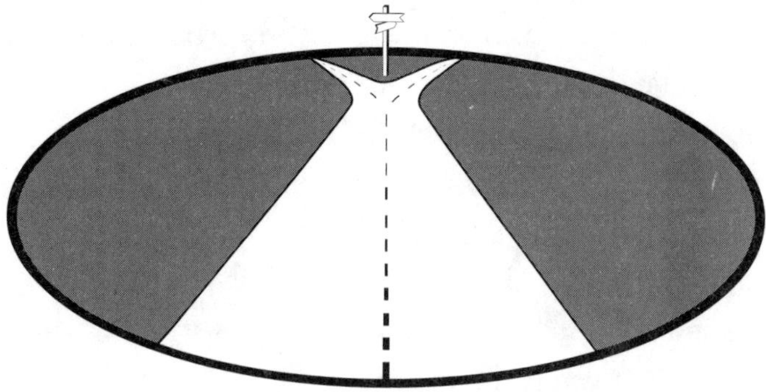

Preparing for the fork in the road

event that patients face a "fork in the road." Most of the testing that is going to be performed has been done already. A decision about bypass surgery or angioplasty has usually already been made, and the necessary procedures completed. At this time, patients face the loss of the comfort and security of being protected and cared for, and need to face the "cold wind" of their independent, formerly active lives. They face the added difficulty of doing so in a weakened state, having gotten "out of shape" because of the forced inactivity after the event, having sustained some amount of heart damage, and having had to take an array of medications that may cause subtle (or not-so-subtle) side effects such as fatigue. No wonder it is tempting to give up!

The silver lining in this apparent dark cloud is that this is the very time that we can make meaningful changes in the way we look at ourselves, the way we behave and the way we react to stresses in our daily lives. Our society, in general, and the structure of medical care in particular, is highly "action-oriented." Caught up in the rush of investigations, treatments and procedures, many patients have little inclination to think seriously about their medical situation. We are constantly surprised that all patients ask "What do I do now?" but very few ever ask "What should I *think* now?" However, as we discuss below, our thoughts and feelings and reactions are very closely related to how the heart behaves, and even related to the risk that we will die. Taking the time for quiet reflection is crucial at this stage. Remember that although heart disease is not your "fault," changing undesirable habits and adopting an optimistic but determined attitude will pay great dividends. Deciding to change your habits and attitudes is the first step to rehabilitation. Research on stopping smoking, for example, indicates that it is very difficult, if not impossible, to stop smoking unless you have decided that you really *want* to stop; if all of the influence comes from outside, for example, from your spouse, family and friends, or from your doctor, this will not be enough to get you to change your behavior in such an important way. This is probably true for all behaviors, whether negative, such as smoking, or positive, such as exercising, improving your diet or adopting a more positive outlook on life. This particular journey requires you to make the decision to actively heal yourself both mentally and physically. Once you have accepted this challenge, which although difficult can be highly rewarding, you will then be able to benefit from the help and support of your loved ones, your doctors, and all those who care for you.

Remember, too, that a lifetime of habits cannot be undone quickly. Fortunately this may not be true for smoking, since most former smokers who quit successfully did so "cold turkey" at the time of an acute event such as a heart attack, usually immediately or very soon after. Precisely how you need to change your habits is discussed in Chapter 6. At this point, we focus on why you should want to change. Having had a heart attack or unstable angina requires some adjustment in everybody. Just as world-class athletes have coaches and trainers, and artistic performers have teachers and directors, all of us can benefit from coaching to learn to deal with our lives in a more positive and healthful way.

Some observations from recent scientific studies help point the way in which this road will take us. Patients who are tired following their heart attacks are more likely to do poorly than are those who are less tired. "Vitality" seems to protect us from cardiac events. Somewhat surprisingly, the severity of the underlying heart disease is not a significant determinant of the amount of fatigue patients experience, suggesting that "tiredness" is a subjective sensation not necessarily related to how hard you have been working or how poor your heart's function is. Many activities, although they involve some effort, may actually help you feel energized, whereas prolonged inactivity, overeating and boredom may actually make you feel "tired," even though you have not really done very much.

Second, those patients who participate in social activities following their heart attacks live longer than those who avoid them. This includes visits with friends; going out to dinner or the theater; or group activities such as club meetings or religious worship. Again, the extent or lack of social participation is not related to the biological seriousness of the heart disease itself, but to other factors that likely include the desire, will and focus to immerse ourselves into our social circle. Such human contact may allow us to look outward instead of focusing on our own troubles and discomforts.

Third, research studies have shown that patients who are "noncompliant" with treatment—in other words, who fail to take their medications as prescribed—have outcomes that are very much worse than those of patients who take their medications faithfully. Not only are effective and beneficial medications not being taken; even patients who do not take their prescribed placebo tablets (an inactive substance) in research studies have higher chances of dying than those who do take their placebo tablets, indicating that the very act of cooperating with medical therapy and believing that the treatment is important enough to warrant continued medication use helps protect against serious, even potentially fatal, heart events.

All of these scientifically based observations imply that a thoughtful decision during recuperation to be actively involved in treatment, to reintegrate back into your social circle, to resume or even expand previous social activities, and to look outward instead of focusing inward is likely not only to help you feel better, but also perhaps to extend your life.

FORUM (MARY): Finding the path of healing

Mary is a fifty-three-year-old single mother of two teenagers whom she had raised alone since early childhood. Mary had recently become more involved with a new boyfriend. There is a strong family history of heart disease on Mary's father's side; she, however, was a nonsmoker, had exercised regularly and had always been well, before she suffered a small heart attack.

Mary was discharged from the hospital without overt complaints, but in the next few weeks she began to experience mild chest tightness and shortness of breath when she was active, which she was almost immediately upon returning home. Activities included her previous exercise routine, work and sex. She was surprised, disappointed and frightened by not being able to "get over it."

Mary was increasingly perplexed that her physical symptoms could not be "solved." She continued trying to go back to work, but kept having a tightness in her chest and shortness of breath climbing stairs at work, and even during meetings. Eventually, she called her cardiologist, complaining, "I'm not getting better and I cannot go on like this." She underwent an exercise test, which showed that her heart muscle was getting insufficient blood supply; and a subsequent angiogram revealed that the blood vessel that had been temporarily blocked, causing her original heart attack, was now quite narrow and almost fully blocked. Angioplasty was recommended and, despite apprehensions and the difficulty of losing further time from her work, she underwent the procedure successfully and was left with moderate heart scarring but no further shortness of breath or chest tightness. She was told to monitor this carefully, and she was placed on drug therapy to lower cholesterol and blood pressure, which she found somewhat of a nuisance. She was also started on an exercise program but was counseled to not overdo physical activities initially, advice which "was against the grain" for somebody who likes to live life at full speed.

In this forum, one year after her heart attack, we invited Mary, her boyfriend and her eighteen-year-old son to discuss this phase of her recovery.

MARY: I'm still confused as to what exactly led to me feeling that I had hit a brick wall after my heart attack. Was it only that my heart was not good, or did I bring it on myself by getting into activities too soon?

DR DORIAN: Your symptoms were not directly caused by overdoing it. Rather, your first heart attack was *incomplete*, and left you at risk for another one. The activity that you tried to do, however, did bring on your chest tightness and shortness of breath, which were signals from your body that your heart was getting insufficient blood and, in turn, meant that you needed further testing and treatment. Although rushing back to your previous life is usually not dangerous, what happened to you highlights the fact that the return to activity needs to be measured, and done in close cooperation with your physician.

MARY: When I think back, it was an unsettled time for me. Strange to say, but once I had been discharged, I just shut my heart out of my mind. I was more concerned that my boyfriend would leave me than anything else.

BOYFRIEND: Well, I hope you have been reassured about that. I was surprised that you could even *think* that I would somehow just abandon you.

MARY: It's easy to look back and say that now, but I didn't know what was going to happen next, especially after my life was so rudely interrupted by my heart. Before that, I had thought I could control everything. After the heart attack, things seemed beyond my control. It was such a relief to know that you were there for me.

SON: You haven't mentioned my sister or me yet. That was a scary time for us too. You weren't well, my dad's been out of the picture for so long now, and we were left to fend for ourselves.

MARY: Yes, those were difficult times for the family.

SON: When you came home the first time, we weren't sure how to handle you, but after only a few days you got busy again.

MARY: You know, I've always solved things that way; only this time, I got a rude shock.

BOYFRIEND: Yes, you found you couldn't do those things you had always done with ease.

MARY: It was a shock when I kept trying and I just couldn't…

Son: Now, Mom, don't get upset.

Mary: Well, I just seemed to hit a brick wall.

Boyfriend: That was when she started to feel down. I had never seen her like that before. You were always such a happy person—so full of energy.

Dr Baker: Yes, Mary, you illustrate well the link between not being able to do something and low mood. When there is the feeling of incapacity, of not feeling capable, which was always so important to you, then instead of feeling on top of the world, the world felt on top of you.

Dr Dorian: Let me jump in here. I can see why you became depressed when you couldn't go back to work or resume your physical activity. However, I think originally this came about because you wanted to deny the fact that you had heart disease. Although dwelling too much on one's heart may not be a good thing, pretending the heart is perfect when it isn't is also not healthy. Many of my patients with a strong family history pretend to ignore (and are sometimes successful at it!) the fact that deep down they are afraid that the same thing that happened to their family members will happen to them. This can result in not seeking or pursuing medical care, and especially not taking medications that are offered or prescribed.

Mary: Well, I can now certainly agree with that. For all those years I didn't want to look at the fact of my family history and I didn't pay much attention to what the doctors told me.

Boyfriend: You mean they found something wrong with you?

MARY: At my regular health checkups I was told that my cholesterol was on the high side. Also, my blood pressure was slightly elevated, but I never pursued any treatment for this.

SON: Mom also never wanted to talk about what had happened with her family…

MARY: I didn't tell you that my father, his brother and my uncle all had heart attacks in their fifties, and my brother has already had bypass surgery.

SON: And that's why, when she had her first attack, my sister and I were very upset.

MARY: I feel now as if I neglected the two of you.

DR BAKER: It looks like you neglected yourself.

SON: Mom, *you* were the one who was ill.

BOYFRIEND: You know, when you first came home from the hospital, you tried to pretend that everything was completely normal, although, of course, I knew it wasn't true. You have always pretended you were invincible, but this time I think you knew that you were in a desperate fight that you thought you could not win. It took you some time to allow me to help you, since I think you felt that this showed that you were weak in some way. I am glad you were eventually able to reach out to me and to your children, who were happy to help you.

DR DORIAN: We find that patients who "bottle up" all of their fears and emotions seem to have more trouble coping than do those who can express their fears and their feelings. In addition, facing up to your fears and recognizing the need for treatment will make it easier for you to follow through with recommendations for medications, tests, and so on, all of which involve a certain amount of nuisance, hassle and possibly discomfort.

MARY: You know, in a sense I think the angioplasty saved my life. That, and that frank discussion I had with my doctor, which made me realize that I was really overdoing things and I needed to slow down and pace myself much better, because things have gone quite smoothly since then.

DR DORIAN: Again, I must point out that "overdoing things" is emotionally unhealthy. However, excessive physical activity is rarely dangerous and simply increases the chance that you develop symptoms such as shortness of breath or chest discomfort. All heart patients have to learn to live within their limitations.

DR BAKER: I gather there have been a number of changes in the family over this time.

SON: Mom was always Supermom until the heart attack. Then, she didn't want us to look after her. But when she found she couldn't do what she wanted to do and she was getting short of breath, she just slowed down; she couldn't help it until she had that procedure.

DR BAKER: What has happened since then?

SON: Mom's different now.

MARY: Also, my healing has turned me around. I'm more open with myself. I don't shut out my problems and I have started to learn to accept help from others. I try to be open with others. I am paying more attention to my children than before. I suppose the family has grown up.

BOYFRIEND: It has changed as well.

MARY: He means that he is also a part of it.

BOYFRIEND: I know that it will take time for me to be fully accepted.

SON: We talked about it and I've told him that we do like him, and we know he's good for Mom.

DR BAKER: A balance is achieved by the end of recuperation, not only in the body and in the mind, but in the family system as well.

MARY: I reckon we are on the way to getting there. Now, I feel more confident, and there is more harmony in the family.

CHAPTER 6

Rehabilitation

rehabilitate: *1. restore to effectiveness or normal life by training etc., esp. after imprisonment or illness* **2.** *restore to former privileges or reputation or a proper condition*

—OXFORD DICTIONARY OF CURRENT ENGLISH

Build me straight, O worthy Master
Staunch and strong, a goodly vessel,
That shall laugh at all disaster,
And with wave and whirlwind wrestle

—H.W. LONGFELLOW

What can Joe do?

Joe's energy was returning step by step; his sleep and appetite were back to normal and he was reading again. What a pleasure! He was starting to feel better. Today, Joe was undergoing evaluation at the rehab center to see whether he was able to exercise vigorously and safely. He wondered if he would pass the test. Weeks ago, he enrolled in a program, but after a few lame attempts at attending, he dropped out. How would he cope with all these activities—the exercise, the lectures and the people? During the dark days of his depression, he had avoided all social contacts. His wife was waiting outside the building, and he didn't want to disappoint her.

We now move on to the more upbeat phase of rehabilitation. Happily, there is a confluence of the restoration of body and mind. Joe has been through his recuperation, when he had to deal with a clinical depression. It is about twelve weeks after his heart attack, and things are now starting to come together for him. He is in the process of getting involved in a supervised program that embodies the hallmark of the rehabilitation process—structured activity. For this phase, we move from the more passive "being" to the active "doing." While rehabilitation takes place along a smoother road, it is not devoid of "bumps," as Joe's story will illustrate. This phase of the journey has its common themes, even though the particulars are different for each patient. We'll conclude this chapter with a discussion with Joe and his wife about rehabilitation, and how Joe has done.

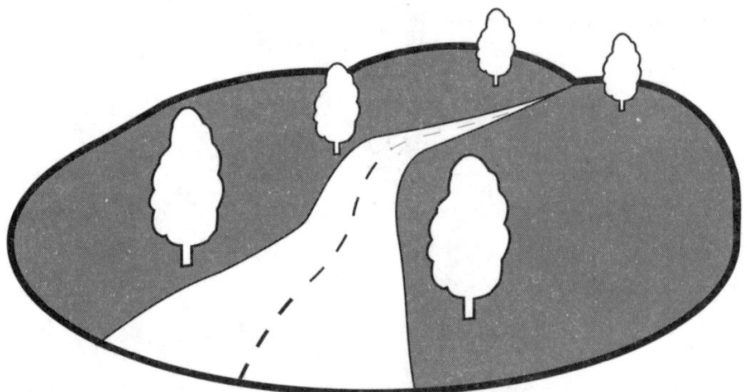

The road of rehabilitation

Rehabilitation has multiple meanings: it is a restoring and active rebuilding of one's health. It implies getting over what you have gone through—the cardiac event and the emotional impact of it. It also means improving your health and well-being, reducing symptoms and even achieving higher fitness levels and more beneficial habits than you had before the event. We want to identify those areas where you need the most attention and individualize rehabilitation for you, as we do not want to run any risk of causing harm. Rehabilitation is usually an upbeat phase: it is positive and forward-looking. And it is strongly linked to activity. This activity is usually structured, and it is the success of programs with structured activities that has helped so many in their journey of recovery.

The exercise aspect of the programs enhances quality of life, improving physical conditioning, which is possible even in the most severely affected patients, gives you more "pep" and allows you to participate in pleasurable activities without fatigue. What is going on at the emotional level during rehabilitation is what others have termed "reconstruction." In Figure 6.1, the circle is being completed. The exposed area which had suffered the impact of the cardiac event is being covered over. This signifies a return to the new "normal" self, which will be heralded by the recovery phase.

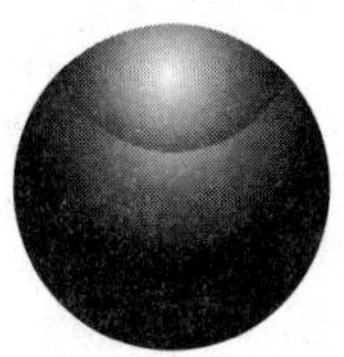

Fig. 6.1
Reconstruction

These days, rehabilitation usually commences in the hospital, with dietary and lifestyle advice, but the supervised programs usually start at about six to eight weeks. From the perspective of the experience of CAD, it is then (about two months after a heart attack) that the emotional stage of reconstruction takes place.

In other fields of recovery, outcome is linked to *structured activity.* The amount and type of activity will depend on the level of physical and emotional function of each individual, but the "programmed," planned, regular aspect of rehabilitation provides the framework that encourages full participation. Work, of course, is itself an activity that is structured, and vocational rehabilitation will also be addressed. Not everyone returns to work, but all patients can participate in some form of program, supervised or not, that has been prescribed by a physician or professional with expertise in this area. Rehabilitation, physical and emotional, takes time—usually a period of several months, at least—and this part of the journey, while a positive one, also has its ups and downs.

Prevention of CAD progression has, as its hallmark, *risk-factor modification.* Risk factors are those diseases, biological properties or habits that increase the chances that CAD will progress or develop. They include high blood cholesterol, smoking, being overweight, physical inactivity, high blood pressure or diabetes, and genetic (inherited) predisposition to CAD. We will naturally have something to say about stress and stress-management programs, which include relaxation techniques as well as anger and time management. Many patients want to know about the intriguing question of stress as the cause of CAD. We are only tentative about making the connection between stress and CAD, not because there is no relationship—there is—but because the connection must be understood in terms of the ubiquitous nature of stress; the degree of risk that it confers, which is usually low; and what we mean by "causation," as opposed to "triggering." (For details, see Part Two, Stress and CAD.)

AN APPROACH TO REHABILITATION

FOR MANY, THE IMAGE that rehabilitation conjures up is of sweatsuited patients jogging around a track, huffing and puffing, and eating raw carrots while they count every calorie. In fact, the recommended regimen may be as simple as taking a brisk walk every day, enjoying what your surroundings have to offer, and slightly altering the kinds of foods that you eat and the size of their portions. The most drastic change required of you during this phase may well be that you consider your body to be your ally, not your enemy. Let your body be your friend and your guide in this journey. The most important trick here is: *listen to your body, but don't be a slave to your body.* Most patients who have a history of heart disease have learned to be very attentive, sometimes too attentive, to the signals that their bodies provide.

Chest tightness or discomfort, dizziness and shortness of breath are very common heart symptoms. Having a past history of these often leads patients to consider, not unreasonably, that any sensations coming from their body are caused by a potentially dangerous heart problem. Most bodily sensations, however, are quite benign. Naturally you will want to check with your doctor to see whether the particular sensations you may be having are important or not. Remember, however, that all of us have aches and pains from time to time, are tired and often don't feel "on top of the world." These feelings are entirely normal. They are particularly common after a heart attack, when you have been inactive, perhaps worried and have to get used to your "new" body, so to speak. *Learning to be comfortable with this new state of affairs* is the first step in your rehabilitation. For example, learn to look upon tiredness as a friend rather than an enemy. If you have taken a walk, or done some other pleasurable activity, expect to be a little tired and use that as a sign that you have helped your body strengthen and heal. If, on the other hand, you are tired after no activity, this may be more a sign of your mood than an indication that your body cannot tolerate activity. Of course, you will want to check with your doctor that any particular activity is safe. In most cases, your body will unambiguously let you know if you have done too much—for example, by becoming quite short of breath. Try not to take your "temperature" too often during this early phase of rehabilitation. If you can get over the initial hump of starting some activity, you will often be pleasantly surprised at how much you can do. Try to go somewhere you will enjoy being, and preferably with a companion so that you can focus on the activity itself rather than on your internal state. Make the activity part of your routine so that it becomes automatic and does not require a renewed decision on each occasion to participate. Remember that rehabilitation is not something that is *done to you*, but something that you *do for yourself*, and for which you can and should take credit.

In his important book *Descartes' Error*, Dr Antonio Damasio explains that the traffic between our brains and our bodies flows both ways, so that our thoughts, moods and emotions are altered by the sensations coming from our bodies and in turn affect our bodily functions, including our hearts. This means that the way in which our brains interpret the signals from our body—for example, pain, fatigue and similar bodily sensations—will influence the way our brains control our bodies. This has two potentially important consequences for patients with heart disease. First, it may mean that part of the benefit of exercise, weight loss, smoking cessation and other healthful habits—in addition to the direct benefits of making the job of the heart easier—may be in preventing unpleasant signal sensations from reaching the brain. When the brain is happier, the heart is happier, as we know from the ill effects of anger on the heart.

Second, we can train our minds to change the interpretation of the signals we receive from our exercising muscles; for example, what was formerly perceived as a sensation of discomfort may be modified to be associated with the positive feeling of strengthening our body and improving our capacity for future activity. Importantly, what used to be thought of as forbidden activity for heart patients is now seen as not only safe, but beneficial. For patients with *congestive heart failure*, a condition in which any form of activity may be difficult, until recently any type of exercise, especially so-called isometric activity (resistance exercise), was seen as prohibited. However, emerging research shows that regular activity such as walking and other forms of light strengthening exercises (e.g., lifting small weights frequently) can significantly improve flexibility, endurance and well-being even in patients with heart failure, who in former years were told "not to lift a finger." In most instances, the body is more resilient than we think, if patients are prepared to put up with the initially unfamiliar sensations of physical effort. The essential part of readying yourself for rehabilitation is the mental preparation for the task, without which the bumps along the road will seem like giant hills—impossible to get beyond.

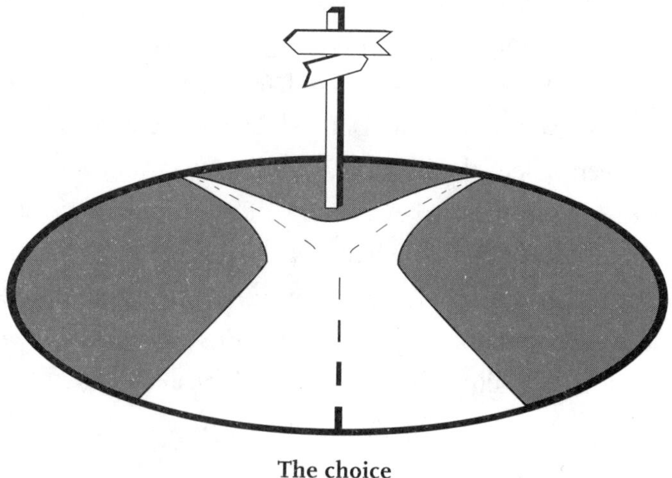

The choice

THE FORK IN THE ROAD

THERE COMES A TIME when the gears can change and the next phase of the journey can begin. How do we know when this is? After the "hurly-burly" of reaction, a state of preparedness is reached. How do we know that we are emotionally ready for reconstruction? The first thing that must be in place is your physical state: your physician has reassured you and declared you stable, whether your symptoms have completely subsided or are still present but are not of serious significance. From the emotional point of view, you will no longer be troubled by anxiety to any prominent degree, and sadness will not dominate, nor low mood weigh you down. Anger will not be a monkey on your back. The appearance of any of these mood states, at times, is normal, and you should not be alarmed by them, but any of these emotional states persisting indicates that a balance has not yet been achieved. The symbol of the fork in the road on the journey of recovery represents the choice that is offered to travelers who are still burdened with residual emotional symptoms. One option is continued reaction. Here, the danger is of continuing a pattern that has become established: we know that habits are hard to break, and the particular habit we want to avoid is the inadvertent establishment of what has been called "the sick role." This occurs in individuals who, though they have received reassurance about their physical state, continue to react and to behave as the "perpetual patient" and retreat into unnecessary dependency. (Note that sometimes—for example, in the situation of a patient like Rose, who is slowly recovering—at least initially, some dependency *is* called for.)

THE IMPORTANCE OF ADAPTIVE DENIAL

FOR DAY-TO-DAY LIVING, what affects our quality of life is the way we are feeling—at the moment. What we are aware of now becomes a crucial factor in our journey of life. We know that in a hundred years' time we will not be around, and in a zillion years our solar system may not exist, but no wonder we choose not to focus on this. After what we have experienced during and after the cardiac event, it would seem natural to want to shut our worries about the future out of our minds, but it is not always easy to do this. During recovery, it is important that we not switch off our minds too much, as this can be to our detriment. In other words, we should not shut out or deny what we *should* be doing to get well. There is an important distinction here—between denial that is "adaptive" and "maladaptive."

Adaptive denial means not being paralyzed by the future. As an example, if we focus on returning to normal immediately, we can be easily overwhelmed, as this rate of recovery is not achievable. If, instead, we focus on small, achievable gains ("I will walk around the block once tomorrow") and disregard for the moment that we are, at present, partially disabled, we are practicing adaptive denial. When Rose does not worry unduly, but follows her treatment regimen, she is engaged in adaptive denial.

If we pretend that all is perfect, that we do not need to make any effort to change any aspect of our lives, we are in *maladaptive denial.* When Tony does not follow his doctor's recommendations and neglects his diet, fails to exercise as he should and resumes smoking, he shows maladaptive denial.

As long as you are following your medical treatment, it is quite acceptable not to focus unduly on your long-term concerns. We say "unduly" because, if you have a particular concern, you should deal with it—just not obsessively. This is where apportionment of time is a judicious thing. In other words, now and then give yourself a break and forget your troubles.

THE MAGIC OF EMPOWERMENT

WATCH THE MOTIVATIONAL speakers on television and you cannot help but be fascinated. The secret of "personal power"! Is it all hokum? Well, we think not. The problem, though, is that, sadly, selling the product (motivational tapes, books, etc.) seems to be the goal. That means a broad market, and little consideration for individual needs and, importantly, individual *timing*. There is no point encouraging you to assert your power when you are not ready for it. If we exhort you to do so at a time when you are still healing, you are going to be very frustrated and disappointed.

Let us take you through the four steps of empowerment. The first step is to *believe* in yourself—start with the belief that you "can do it" if you put your mind to it. The next step is to *determine* what you are able to do, basing your judgment on the advice and information you have obtained. Third, cautiously proceed to *demonstrate* what you can do. The final step is *mastery*—the capability or skill of being able to do it. What we are describing has been found to enhance your recovery—namely, "self-efficacy," or the belief that you are *effective* in what you do. Once you have been through the four-step sequence, you will feel the magic of empowerment, a key ingredient of the reconstruction component of rehabilitation.

THE SECRET OF EMPOWERMENT: STRUCTURED ACTIVITY

WHAT IS THE MEDIUM through which "empowerment" occurs? There is no point giving you an abstract noun (empowerment) and expecting that this, in itself, is the solution. As Wittgenstein, the famous philosopher, discovered, it is not the direct meaning of the word that is important, but the use to which the word is put. The reason that empowerment "takes" during rehabilitation is that we are ready for it and, furthermore, there is an ideal context in which to use it. This context has two components:

the first is graded *activity*; the second is the *structured* nature of the activity. Given the cardiac event that has occurred, it is necessary to have *professional direction* as to what structured activity we are able to do. It is for this reason that the ideal setting initially is a *supervised* one. Traditionally, such supervision involves direct observation, such as at a rehabilitation research center in a hospital or freestanding dedicated facility. Recent research has shown that rehabilitation "at home" with regular if infrequent phone calls from a rehab "case worker" can be just as effective in maintaining an exercise regimen and heart-healthy habits. In our opinion, most patients find it difficult to adhere to a program "at a distance." The incentive that comes with regular, scheduled attendance at a clinic, and the social contact and support that come from participating in group activities more than compensate for the inconvenience of the travel involved.

The success of rehabilitation programs is attested to by the recent increases in the number of programs available. The importance of the key ingredients of education, supervised individualized exercise programs and, finally, the social contacts afforded should not be underestimated. Structured activity is a prescribed component of the programs and, as the activity is performed and goals are reached, *mastery* occurs. We discussed how, during the reaction phase, low mood is associated with not being able to *do* things. This is a natural relationship. When things are "on top" of you, you feel down. When you feel "on top of the world," this means that you are happy. With mastery comes the sense of accomplishment that can put you there.

Work: The ultimate structured activity?

Now, back to the real world... The programs don't take up most of your time, and they also don't go on forever, usually lasting up to a year. Also, in the real world, many have to earn a living. When it comes to work, there may be the risk of "too much of a good thing"—too much activity and too much structure. Thus, vocational rehabilitation can be a key component in the recovery process.

We know that some of those who have had a cardiac event will simply not be able to work—ever (see Rose), at first (see Joe)—or are pushing too strongly to work at the wrong time (see Mary), a type of maladaptive denial. Many patients will be able to return to work, but not all continue to do the same work they did before.

A graded approach to work eligibility is usually required. The question of disability—full-time or part-time, with respect to one's own job or any job—is complicated by the issue of compensation. If the decision is made by a third party (for example, an insurance company), unfortunately an adversarial situation is often created, in which one party is attempting to disprove something, and another to prove something—and the truth is often in the middle! On the one hand, disability payment can act as an incentive to further improvement and provide important coverage for those who cannot work. On the other, the protection of financial support and the perceived stresses of returning to a job can be a disincentive to plunging back into the competitive world of work. Of course, this is a gray area, and often the emotional side comes into play. In many situations suitability for work becomes a matter of opinion, although some disorders, such as clinical depression, make the decision quite clear. To avoid too much complexity, then, we state the obvious: "You can only do what you can do!" However, even this advice is not entirely straightforward, as you must consider "what you can do." A combination of objective opinion, honest subjective appraisal and a phased approach is in the patient's best interest in deciding about returning to work.

CAN I PREVENT MY CAD FROM RECURRING OR PROGRESSING?

CARDIAC REHABILITATION USUALLY focuses on the major *risk factors* for coronary artery disease. These include elevated cholesterol, smoking, high blood pressure, diabetes, obesity, physical inactivity and perhaps certain personality profiles. A family history of coronary heart disease, especially in close relatives who were diagnosed with heart disease before age sixty-five, indicates that you are at increased risk of developing coronary disease yourself—but of course this particular risk cannot be modified. Recent theories, yet to be proven, suggest that hardening of the arteries may have as a contributing factor inflammation of the artery wall indirectly caused by a chronic infection potentially treatable with antibiotics. In addition, higher amounts than normal of a substance called homocysteine in the blood can increase the risk of heart attacks. This factor may be important since it can be mitigated with a vitamin-like food constituent called folic acid.

It must be emphasized that, for most patients, no single or combination of risk factors is known to be *the* cause of heart disease. Many people in fact have no risk factors for coronary artery disease, and thus may legitimately ask, "Why me?", having perceived themselves as having done "nothing wrong." Although statistics tell us that risk factors, especially combinations of risk factors, do indeed increase the *likelihood* that someone will develop hardening of the arteries, our ability to predict in given individuals how likely they are to develop heart disease or a worsening of heart disease is not very good. Rehabilitation therefore must focus on a general approach to diminishing all possible risk factors.

A great deal has been written about proper nutrition, particular exercise programs and stopping smoking. No one particular diet, exercise program or approach to stopping smoking is right for all individuals. Every person has his or her own unique profile of circumstances, needs and opportunities to which a particular rehabilitation program needs to be adapted. The best programs will thus deal with each person as an individual, and tailor a "made-to-measure" program that fits his or her own particular style and possibilities. For example, a program of long-distance walking may not be applicable in communities where the winters are long and where there are no indoor facilities for exercise. A diet emphasizing fresh fruits and vegetables, which is highly desirable, may be inappropriate for individuals with financial difficulties, or in communities where some of these items may be in short supply in the winter. As we emphasized above, perhaps the most important aspect of rehabilitation is assisting the patient to come to terms with the need for self-assessment and need to choose a positive, optimistic road toward improved well-being. Beginning the rehabilitation program with calm, contemplative decision making is essential if the program is to succeed and be maintained in the long run.

Patients often ask, "How do I stop smoking?" or "How do I begin an exercise program?" We always answer: "First you have to *want* to do it." In other words, you have to make an active decision to break a bad habit or develop a good one of your own free will and with a positive resolve. Once you have taken that step, actually doing what is required is little more than a detail.

FAMILY CONCERNS

IT IS FAIR TO SAY that the rehabilitation phase is usually an easier time for patient and family—certainly, as compared with the previous phases. By now, a balance in the family will have been established, but it may still take some time, maybe months, for a new, steady equilibrium within the family system to emerge. There will be times when the patient is dependent on the spouse as he or she progresses; as well, there will be the normal ups and downs of their journey, and there may well be "slippage" (see page 112). Even so, for most, further recovery can be expected.

Your support is helpful to the patient, but are you supported yourself? You can benefit from the information exchange and camaraderie of time-limited educational group sessions offered to patients and their families. Finding out what can help you is particularly pertinent to those spouses or significant others who have taken more of the emotional brunt than the patient. You can decide whether intervention (say, counseling) may benefit you (see Part Two).

There may be questions of whether you can resume all aspects of your married life, especially those with which you were happy and that stopped because of the cardiac event. Attending a follow-up doctor's appointment with the patient can be an invaluable way to restore and maintain the balance in the marital relationship, and, consequently, in the family as well (assuming doctor and patient give permission for you to be there).

Family relationships are dynamic; they change, and different members can be affected at different times by what is happening to the patient, especially in the early stages, but also later, as slippage can occur. Much will depend on the flexibility of the family system before the event. If it tended to be shaky then, it will be after a cardiac event as well, but by the time the patient is engaged in active rehabilitation, the restabilization of the family should already be well under way.

Family members as well as patients should be aware of what the patient *and* they themselves go through. They may also benefit from stress-management techniques: the "Ten Commandments of stress management" (below) apply to them as well as to patients. Parents should be on the lookout for untoward behavior by children, who often display their emotional problems in unexpected ways. If there is a suspicion of an underlying problem, a professional should be consulted. As a spouse, you will be expected to be involved in the recovery of the patient, and you will have met the specialists and family doctor. You may also want to participate in group educational sessions that are now often included as part of informational sessions after a cardiac event or are optional in rehab programs.

We would be remiss if we failed to mention *Heartmates*, the book, video and organization created by Rhoda Levin, a spouse who experienced her husband's heart attack and realized the insufficiency of support systems for caregivers. These materials are helpful in understanding what the spouse goes through and what can be done about it. (See "Recommended Reading.")

A GUIDE TO THE REHAB PROGRAMS

CARDIAC REHABILITATION INVOLVES restoring patients to the best possible cardiac health, which includes the ability to perform physical activities; reduce risk factors for coronary heart disease; and encourage the best possible social, psychological and vocational functioning. In practice, this means enabling patients to do the physical and social activities that they would like to be able to do, without symptoms, and to minimize any psychological distress that may come from having had a recent cardiac event.

Traditional rehabilitation programs usually emphasize the exercise component. They usually involve supervised, or at least guided, programs of approved regular physical activity, done at an intensity that is believed to be safe. *Isotonic exercise* involves using large muscle groups such as the legs or arms to move the body through space. Activities such as walking, jogging, swimming and bicycling are examples of isotonic exercise. If done frequently enough (three or more times per week) and long enough (thirty minutes or longer), this type of exercise will increase cardiovascular fitness. Fitness is the ability to do physical activity and derives from increased efficiency on the part of exercising muscles. The heart does not actually become stronger with regular activities, but the body, and especially the exercising muscles, can learn to use the blood and oxygen provided by the heart more efficiently with training. Exercise produces impressive gains with only a moderate amount of effort, provided that the exercise is of sufficient duration and frequency to get a training effect. Heart patients do not need to become competitive athletes in order to benefit from exercise programs; rather, they need to have the desire and the will to maintain a program that can be of surprisingly low intensity (for example, modestly brisk, continuous walking) and that is often pleasurable (think of a walk through your neighborhood, in a nearby park, with the companionship of a loved one or a friend, or perhaps a pet), and can lead to increases in well-being. Even patients with very poor heart function, so-called heart failure, will derive some benefit from physical activity, allowing them to do more, with less distress, although they may not be restored to complete heart health.

Another recommended form of exercise is *isometric exercise*, performed by straining or pushing against resistance. This includes lifting weights; calisthenics such as sit-ups; and floor exercises such as gymnastics, yoga or tai chi. In all of these forms of exercise work, muscles are made to contract against resistance, and thereby become stronger; although it used to be thought that such forms of exercise might be dangerous for heart patients, we now know that they can increase strength, endurance, flexibility and well-being even in elderly patients with severe heart disease. Of course, this type of exercise needs to be done with proper technique and only after instruction from an expert.

These activities need not be done at an intensity that is painful or uncomfortable. The adage "no pain, no gain" is sometimes used by athletes training for competitive events. This is definitely not true for cardiac patients; in fact, the kinds of activities that can lead to a training effect and increase well-being are often gentle enough to be enjoyable and pleasurable while producing only minimum fatigue or shortness of breath. What is crucial for patients embarking on these programs is to learn to enjoy the feeling of exercising the body and the feeling of movement that goes along with the particular activity.

Another important component of rehabilitation programs is modifying behavior to minimize the impact of risk factors for heart disease, and educating patients about their illness and how to reduce their chances of having future events. Risk factors known to predispose to coronary heart disease (hardening of the arteries), or to the likelihood of a recurrent event, are by now well known to most readers, and include high cholesterol in the blood, cigarette smoking, diabetes, high blood pressure, obesity, certain kinds of personality or behavioral style, and genetic or inherited predispositions. The good news is that risk factors, other than genetic ones, *can* be changed, with behavior modification or with medication, or both, and that changing these risk factors can undoubtedly have a beneficial impact on the risk of future events as well as on well-being.

Although changing one's attitude and behavior on one's own definitely can modify some of these risk factors, especially those involving diet, stopping smoking and exercise, for most patients professional help, and often medications, are required.

A detailed discussion of the importance of and different kinds of cholesterol (the "good," the "bad" and the "ugly") is beyond the scope of this book. It is very important to remember, however, that most individuals find lowering their blood cholesterol through diet alone extremely difficult. In our experience, achieving a change in diet is more a matter of changing your philosophy toward eating than of knowing what foods to eat and what foods to avoid, or "dieting," in the sense of depriving yourself of food. This includes learning how to enjoy the flavor of low-fat foods, for example, spices, herbs, fruits and vegetables, and learning to listen carefully to the signals of hunger and fullness by which your body tells you whether it is time to eat or not. Our North American lifestyle, with television watching, spectator sports and social activities centered around drinking alcohol and eating high-fat foods, is not conducive to heart-healthy habits. In this sense, the best steps to improving your diet may be to watch less television and to engage in more outdoor activities, where you are less likely to snack.

Drugs to lower cholesterol are very effective, are known to prolong life and are quite safe, although they may be a nuisance to take regularly and are not inexpensive. There should be no shame in taking medications to lower cholesterol, since even extraordinarily strict diets achieve only modest cholesterol lowering in most patients. Similarly, high blood pressure and diabetes respond well to drug treatment but cannot be cured (although they *can* be helped) by diet and exercise. An active decision to work with your doctors and caregivers to follow a treatment plan is very important, both since it will help you achieve your goals and since a positive attitude toward your treatment will be, in and of itself, beneficial.

Probably the most important, but often ignored, aspect of cardiac rehabilitation is increasing *knowledge* so that patients understand precisely what is happening to their bodies, and the benefits of the changes that they, together with their doctors, can bring about. Understanding the benefits (the *why*) as well as the details (the *what*) of rehabilitation can change it from "work," like a school assignment, to a pleasurable activity that is done for its own sake as well as to improve heart health. Your most important task as a heart patient is to come to terms with this need to understand your heart, your body and your mind, and to work on this attitude, which requires you to see yourself not as a victim, but as a mind/body system that can powerfully influence your heart's future. If there is any aspect of your heart health that you do not understand, be sure to ask it of your caregivers, and accept an answer only if you understand it completely.

Rehabilitation is not something that you just do for a few weeks or a few months after a heart event. Unfortunately, coronary artery disease can never be completely reversed. You therefore need to continue on your journey indefinitely, always aware that you have some small risk of a repeat heart event, but that this risk can be managed and controlled by continuously taking care of yourself and keeping up a vigilant attitude. Remember that it took twenty or thirty years for the hardening of the arteries to develop, and that your habits of living have evolved slowly since your childhood. Don't be too hard on yourself, therefore, and don't expect that you can change either your heart vessels or your heart habits overnight. As you gradually learn new habits, they will become second nature. Nevertheless, much in the way that anything in life that is worth having requires dedication and effort, maintaining heart-healthy habits requires a continuous and conscientious commitment. This need not be painful or distressing, but maintaining a positive attitude and beneficial changes in your diet and activity will not happen automatically. This is especially true with respect to your attitude toward yourself and your illness. Much as anger obstructs your path to recovery, and passivity leads to paralysis, equanimity combined with a realistic but determined attitude can help you deal with the inevitable frustrations of everyday life that all of us face.

The Ten Commandments of stress management

Most of us could use some stress management. We take stress so much for granted that we are unaware of the load that is accumulating on us. We don't want you to be like Humpty Dumpty; we want you to feel "together," as they say. In Part Two, we describe the vulnerabilities to stress and the methods to overcome them. Here, we offer these "commandments" in a lighthearted way that we hope will not offend or be otherwise stressful to you!

1. ***Thou shalt expect stress and, when it does occur, thou shalt not overreact.***

   Demands are part of life. As is so well-articulated in the book *The Road Less Traveled* (by M. Scott Peck), the wisdom of this statement is in realizing that since stress is to be expected, we can deal with it better if we are not surprised or upset every time things don't go our way. Many people thrive on stress, as long as it doesn't overwhelm them. At the other end of the spectrum are those who are sensitive to each stressor as it occurs. They have difficulty filtering out unnecessary stimuli. For those who are sensitive to the environment, life has a decidedly "jumpy" quality, since with sensitivity comes reactivity. Such people respond to problems with an intensity that in and of itself serves to heighten the negative experience and cause further problems. In the context of CAD, a vicious circle can result when anxiety and physical symptoms such as chest pain interact (see page 207). Thus, overreacting will increase your distress.

   When an obviously stressful event occurs, a response is inevitable, and you should take time to recover. This book describes the phased response to a cardiac event. By now, you are very familiar with what you can expect when this type of trauma occurs. This sequence of responses can be modified to apply to most stressors and the impact such events have on us and our loved ones. By being familiar with what may happen, we are more able to formulate a normal response to an abnormal occurrence. It would be helpful for us to be familiar with our own responses, so that we "go easy" on ourselves during the vulnerable phases and are able to forge ahead at the appropriate time for reconstruction.

2. *Thou shalt eliminate stress that is ongoing and too demanding.* It is common for us to get into unhealthy patterns in our everyday lives, such as job and marriage. We adjust to the level of stress, but often this level is much higher than what is healthy for us. The metaphor of riding a horse is a useful way to look at how you deal with your life. When the horse is standing still, there is no problem staying on. As he starts to walk, there is still no problem. A canter is a pleasure; faster, and there is the thrill of riding. However, we all concede that there is a certain point beyond which only an experienced rider should venture. Go even further, and you have a rodeo on your hands, and you *will* be thrown. Many people spur themselves on to a dangerous extent. Once thrown, fight or flight will take place—anger or fear—and, if this persists, low mood will result. We are riding the horse in too charged a way. If we are comfortably riding at a trot, we should easily be able to handle any eventuality. So, we need to deal with the overburdensome areas of our lives in ways that are constructive, and to generally pace ourselves so that stress is manageable and the consequent distress minimal.

3. *Thou shalt follow doctors' orders: prescribed exercise is good stress management!* Patients who follow doctors' orders, including the regular taking of medication, will run into fewer problems than those who

do not. One of the reasons for good cardiac outcome is the increasingly better control medications give us over symptoms. The body's ability to improve in terms of residual cardiac function has been greatly enhanced by new developments in medical treatment. We have described the benefits of the exercise component of the rehabilitation programs. In addition, exercise functions as a type of stress management. It is a "burn-off" approach, as opposed to the "calm down" approach of the stress-management programs. Not following your prescribed treatment is usually detected at follow-up, and this breeds mistrust, which undermines the previously solid edifice of the relationship with your doctor. Remember, you never know when you will need your doctor—she or he could save your life!

4. *Thou shalt get a professional evaluation if distress persists.*
Even books like this have their shortcomings! We hope to open up your minds (and hearts) to what happens and to what you can do to enhance recovery from a cardiac event. But we cannot expect you to diagnose yourself; as we have said before, if your symptoms are severe and/or persistent, seek professional advice. This book is not designed to tell you all there is to know about each evaluation, including clinical depression. We are merely increasing awareness. So, remember, when in doubt, seek a professional out!

5. *Thou shalt identify thy needs and practice stress-management techniques regularly, wherever and whenever you must.*
What do you need? If things are going along quite well, you may not need any extra programs. But recently there has been more interest in stress-management techniques. Should everyone use them? We think not; but many *could* benefit from them. Herbert Benson described the mental and physical effect

of the "relaxation response," which occurs after relaxing in a specific, focused way. Two components characterize the techniques that elicit the response. One we can call "focusing"; the other, "defocusing." The truth is, it's not really that difficult. By focusing the mind, the response can be achieved, on the condition that all other incoming stimuli, such as thoughts and images, are pushed aside. After a short time, the recognizable response of relaxation is experienced.

There are two approaches to teaching relaxation—the group and the individual method. For most patients, we recommend the group method supervised by *experienced* group teachers. However, the person who has identifiable symptoms of anxiety derives a better result from the individual method. The techniques are *deep breathing*, *progressive muscular relaxation*, *autogenic relaxation*, *imaging* and *meditation*. Patients usually do not like all the techniques equally. You must find out what works for you and then use it. We recommend active rather than passive methods (such as audiotapes), unless you cannot do it for yourself. Patients should practice relaxation techniques with the same frequency as they exercise, that is, at least three or four times per week. They will then develop an expertise in "turning on" the technique, and will be better able to use it when necessary in "real life" situations (see Part Two).

In contrast to those who experience anger as a temporary emotional reaction to the cardiac event ("Why me?"), those who have *ongoing* problems with anger—be it thinking, feeling or expressing it—will need anger-management techniques. If there is a strong arousal (feeling "overalert") component with associated anxiety, relaxation techniques are also useful. For someone who has reported negative thinking linked to anger, cognitive psychotherapy can be helpful. The group setting can be invaluable to patients with anger problems. As with all group treatment, the group *must* be led by an experienced group leader. (For general information see *Anger Kills* by R. and V. Williams.)

Over the years physicians have observed how cardiac patients seem to be pressured by time. Psychologists have developed elaborate methods to determine if you suffer from "time urgency," such as feeling hurried or doing more than one thing at a time. Although the link to cardiac outcome is not clear, it seems that certain individuals can benefit from training in time management, by getting their lives into balance and by handling stress more competently. Many people are time-pressured at work; even if, as they often say, "that's part of the job description," changes are needed. Time pressure, anger and impaired stress management are often linked. For example, if people who are always in a rush take on "one more problem" or run into "one more thing," the house of stress cards may collapse! Such people need to be aware that there is too much time pressure in their lives (see Part Two).

6. ***Thou shalt look on the bright side.***
You will have a head start in dealing with stress if you can learn to think positively. The way you perceive events can be as significant to your quality of life as the events themselves. Studies now suggest that a favorable disposition can improve your health outcome. We take the way we look at the world for granted—that's the way it is. Not so! Experience can mold your outlook in a positive or negative way. The pessimist will draw up a long list showing how badly life has treated them, with the cardiac event as further proof. But if you adjust your lenses to perceive the world in a more positive light, the experience can have a different meaning for you. For example, the cardiac event could be seen as a warning to you to live your life in a different way—in a sense it has "saved your life."

The optimist accepts stress and deals with it. A positive and realistic interpretation of the stressful event will allow you to handle stress better and your heart health will benefit as well. And your pleasant disposition will be attractive to others, providing you with more support. By looking on the bright side, you will feel better.

7. *Thou shalt try to have a spiritual side.*
We have come to appreciate, and now the research is starting to confirm, that having a spiritual underpinning to one's outlook in life is a great aid to recovery. It doesn't seem to matter what you believe in as long as you have a belief system. Science helps us to explain measurable phenomena, and there is an explosion of such knowledge in all areas. But the deeper questions remain completely unexplained. A belief system gives us meaning and allows us to trust in the world around us. When the belief system is in the form of organized religion, the structure and comfort of rituals and communal prayer also help to sustain people. Additionally, the benefits of the social aspects of fellowship and community should not be understated. In whatever form, meaningful rituals, prayer, and especially a belief system, can be sustaining in the recovery from a cardiac event and seems generally good for your health.

8. *Thou shalt have a good support system.*
Having good support from the people around you is a favorable factor for cardiac outcome. Precisely what component of social support is the helpful part has not yet been determined, but intimate relationships, close friendships and other social networks have been examined, and, for your purposes, we can simply state that good social support is a healthy thing.

There is nothing as strong and as helpful as a supportive spouse. But for those not in an intimate relationship, the presence of supportive close friends or family serves a similar function. Even a circle of supportive acquaintances is very helpful, especially when you enjoy their company and the contact is quite frequent. Rehabilitation programs and religious congregations can also provide the social support component, in addition to other obvious benefits.

9. ***Thou shalt not be stressed by the stress-management programs!*** A strange phenomenon encountered by many cardiac patients (and others too) is the stress that is produced by the need to do well in stress-management programs. More and more techniques and programs are being offered, and many people feel they *must* do exactly what is prescribed. We cannot believe in "all fits one and one fits all." You must *individualize your program* and realize that not every instruction applies to you. Similarly, "busy" patients who rush around trying to squeeze programs into their already frenzied schedules are on a treadmill of futility, defeating the purpose of the exercise! Finally, some patients succumb to the phenomenon of "life as therapy," where one's whole life is taken over by various programs and their activities. We would not interfere with people who are devoted to the cause in such a single-minded way: their belief in their system is an added benefit. For most, though, it is simply not necessary to go to such extremes.

10. ***Thou shalt seek out humor. No kidding.*** Finally, there is no more pleasant admonition than to ask you to look for the humor in your life. Humor and laughter are wonderful safety valves installed in our brains. There are even

humor therapists now, but we think that this is a bit of a joke! Unfortunately, not everyone is equally lighthearted, but all can learn to see the funny side of things. People will be surprised by how much laughing goes on behind the therapist's door, but care must be taken that humor is not being used as a defense against issues that need to be discussed seriously or as an outlet for underlying angry feelings. The ability to find the humorous side, when life is difficult, is something for which we must keep searching.

SLIPPAGE

As sure as day follows night, so our journey has ups and downs. When we have worked hard in rehabilitation, and expect a smooth road to recovery, we can be severely disappointed if we do hit a bumpy patch. As in all aspects of life, improvement or progress after an event is not steady. Weeks or months of getting better can be interrupted by a temporary halt in progress, or even a setback. These are normal and do not mean that you will slip back to where you were just after the event.

Once you have been treated, the risk of an event recurring in the short term is significantly reduced, but not eliminated. If symptoms or events do occur, you must deal with them! Part Two outlines what to do in an emergency, but the main direction is pretty simple: if you are not sure, seek expert help! Otherwise, there is no need to be in a state of heightened alert; emotionally it is not good for you.

By now you will have established a network of professionals whom you trust and who are accessible to you. Whether the issue in question is of heart or of mind, consult an expert. If emotional symptoms recur, try to identify them: this alone can sometimes help to resolve things; use what you know. Or calmly discuss the problem with a confidante who has the objectivity to help you or advise you. But if the problem is persistent, seek professional advice; often simple counseling or the reinforcement of what you already know will help to remedy the situation. It is useful to remind ourselves that we are never able to predict actual incidents, but we are able to see trends, and, importantly, we are able to deal with any eventualities.

Another form of slippage is not complying with your treatment recommendations. This can occur almost without being noticed, but if you are not consistently modifying the risk factors—that is, eating healthy, exercising appropriately, avoiding smoking and, of course, taking your medications—you will be "stacking the odds" against a good recovery and increasing the chances of a recurrent cardiac event.

So far, this book has attempted to increase awareness so as to promote a better recovery. The "carrot and stick" approach is a pretty effective motivator. The "stick" has been mentioned: poorer outcome. The carrot is the converse: a better outcome and, importantly, a good quality of life. We highlight how to integrate healthy heart habits and an enjoyable quality of life in the next chapter, when we discuss the "challenge of maintenance."

FORUM (JOE): Getting into gear

Joe is a sixty-three-year-old accountant who has mild diabetes and is slightly overweight. He has never smoked and, aside from being inactive, has been, as far as he was concerned, in good health all his life. So, when he suffered a fairly large heart attack, it came as a complete surprise to him. Although he had no complications in the hospital and was able to do an exercise test on the treadmill quite well before going home, he never really was able to resume his former activities.

He didn't have side effects from the medications, and didn't have shortness of breath or chest pain or dizziness, even with climbing stairs or walking briskly. However, he could never get his motivation or energy high enough to want to go out, go for walks or attend social events with his family and friends; he also completely lost interest in sex. Although he went back to work, he found himself staring out the window and unable to concentrate. Rehabilitation was recommended, but he found the appointments difficult to manage and attended sessions only once in a while. He really didn't feel like driving for thirty minutes in order to put shorts and a t-shirt on and walk around a small track with other heart-attack victims.

It was only when Joe's business partner was reminded of his own brother's depression that the "penny dropped" and he called Joe's wife. Soon thereafter, a clinical depression was diagnosed, and Joe was started on antidepressant treatment, as well as given supportive psychotherapy; his wife attended sessions as well.

Soon Joe's mood lifted considerably, his motivation returned, he began to be interested in the world around him and he was able to eventually start the rehabilitation program. For the first few months of rehabilitation, Joe had no major problems.

Joe attended this forum with his wife, Dr Baker and Dr Dorian.

Joe: I found a lot of things to interest me in this particular chapter, although personally I think that most of the drama for myself had occurred in the previous phase. Rehabilitation itself went quite smoothly.

Wife: Not the first time you tried to join the program.

Joe: I was depressed at the time. I wonder how many others are dropping out for that or other reasons.

Dr Baker: After heart attack there are about one-third of patients who have some form of depression and this could well affect compliance. Also, there are those people who live far away from the rehab programs, those who get involved in work commitments and also those who shut their minds off from their having heart disease (what we called "maladaptive denial"). These people probably don't want to face up to the challenge of what it means to have heart disease.

Joe: Well, I can sympathize with those who have been depressed, especially all those people who don't even know about it.

Wife: You talked about work commitments. I think Joe doesn't admit to how much work he takes on.

Joe: I do what I have to do.

Wife: We have discussed this many times. When it comes to sharing the work, Joe always lands up with the lion's share. It's been going on for years.

Joe: It's true that I have trouble saying no.

Wife: Yes, you're always "Mr Nice Guy." Remember, "nice guys finish last."

Dr Baker: If you are not assertive, you may be taken advantage of, even though your partners may not be aware that they are overloading you and don't mean any harm to you.

Joe: No, they don't. They were wonderful to me when I was not up doing things after the heart attack, and especially when it turned out that I was depressed.

Wife: You were delayed in starting the rehab program the second time, but we were just relieved that you were feeling well. In the end it doesn't seem to have mattered so much as long as you eventually did what you had to do.

Dr Dorian: Joe, I understand that you developed problems later on.

Joe: Well, I had no problems at first, but it must have been about six months after the heart attack, I suddenly became dizzy and my heart started to pound. This went on for half an hour. I went to my doctor and he said that my heartbeat was irregular. I had to wear a Holter monitor and, during that time, I had a bout of palpitations, recorded on the monitor, which they later told me was "atrial fibrillation."

Dr Dorian: This is a form of heart rhythm disturbance, or arrhythmia, which is non–life threatening but can be problematic. The good thing is that it can be effectively treated with drugs.

JOE: Yes, once they got the right combination of my medications, I have stayed well ever since.

DR DORIAN: How did you handle it compared with the heart attack?

JOE: Well, it was completely different! When I first had the heart attack, I felt completely at a loss. I thought my life was basically over, even though I realized somehow that I could still function physically. I felt guilty at not having taken better care of myself with regard to my diet, not having exercised more, not having watched my diabetes more carefully. I just couldn't motivate myself to go to the exercise classes because I just couldn't see any point in going through all that if it wasn't going to help me. When the doctors would explain things to me, I don't think I was really listening, because I thought it was really hopeless. A few weeks after I started taking the medication for depression, I began to see that I wasn't quite so sick as I had feared, and that if I participated fully in the program it could help me. Only then did I find that I could exercise, and concentrate on my work, and began to be much more hopeful that I would continue to improve.

WIFE: He's asking you about how you handled the arrhythmia.

JOE: Sorry. So, as I was saying, when the atrial fibrillation suddenly happened, I discovered I had confidence and I wasn't devastated by it. I am sure that had I had the arrhythmia earlier after the heart attack, the dizziness and the heart irregularity would have made me think I was dying, that my life was in danger.

Dr Baker: For you, the decision to move on on the road of rehabilitation was easy, once your depression lifted. It is not always so easy for others. As a cardiologist, what do you do, Dr Dorian, to motivate patients after a heart event, those not clinically depressed?

Dr Dorian: I think getting patients to go even once to the program, just to try it out, can give a boost. Once patients see how helpful the staff are, that they are not alone, and that others have taken the same route and done well, they can see a light on the horizon.

Dr Baker: Joe, what was your experience of the supervised program like?

Joe: After I began the rehab program, although I must say I wasn't very optimistic about it in the beginning, I gradually began to get some pep and energy back, and I could see how it could help me. I was also able to listen more carefully to my doctor and follow the coaches in the program. The good news is that the better I felt, the more eager I got; and the more I did, the better I felt. I began to look forward eagerly to my three-times-a-week sessions at the rehab center and was even able to help convince some of my fellow patients that they should hang in there with the program.

Wife: I must say it was a pleasure to see how enthusiastic he became with the program. He was also very strict when it came to cutting down on the fats in his diet and continuing to exercise religiously.

Joe: Well, it seemed to give me more meaning in my life. Sticking to the diet took some getting used to, but I like my wife's cooking, whatever she makes.

WIFE: I think Joe is flattering me to keep me cooking up a storm for the next few years!

DR DORIAN: What about exercise?

JOE: Being at the program really helped me get used to doing exercise. I feel good during and also after I have completed my prescribed program.

WIFE: Joe, don't you think you became so much better when you met your friend over there?

JOE: That's right. You know, even though I had been down in the dumps and not very keen, when Fred came into the program, I felt so good being able to convince him of the benefits of the program. As time went on, we saw that we had a lot in common and became good friends. We encourage each other driving together to the rehab center, discussing our diets and walking together.

DR BAKER: One cannot overestimate the value of friendship and generally the social aspects of rehabilitation programs. This certainly seems to have given an impetus to you, Joe, in helping you along the road to recovery. What about your handling of stress?

JOE: From what I've read here, I think I'm okay.

WIFE: You still haven't stopped taking on too much work.

DR BAKER: Well, if this continues, I suggest you do assertiveness training.

WIFE: As long as he is not like that at home!

Dr Baker: I know that you are joking, but learning how to stick up for yourself and being firmer with others will extend to all areas.

Wife: I think I can handle that. I'm only too pleased that Joe is getting his life in order.

Joe: My wife hasn't mentioned how wonderfully supportive she has been. She has helped me so much. Things look so different at the end of rehabilitation, compared to the beginning of it!

CHAPTER 7

Recovery

recover 1. regain possession, use or control, 2. return to health, consciousness, or to a normal state or position

—Oxford Dictionary of Current English

All's well that ends well.

—Shakespeare

Has Kevin recovered?

Sometimes, when Kevin thought of all that that taken place over the past year it was still hard to recall the events surrounding his unexpected surgery without getting upset. The first days and weeks had been quite a strange experience, and difficult for his wife as well. Then he had felt unsettled. But lately he had been feeling quite well. He had never been so physically fit! It was a bit of a grind, but he was sticking to his dietary program.

Kevin couldn't change his temperament though. Small things would still set him off; he could get upset quite easily and, in certain circumstances, he still had a temper. But he understood the need to reflect and not to react, and for the most part he controlled himself. He was a calmer man than before this heart thing had emerged. What had happened had changed his wife too. She had learned to handle crises better than before. Adversity had strengthened the marriage. Both of them understood and accepted that he was a "heart patient," but that, first and foremost, he was Kevin, and they were ready to move on to other journeys.

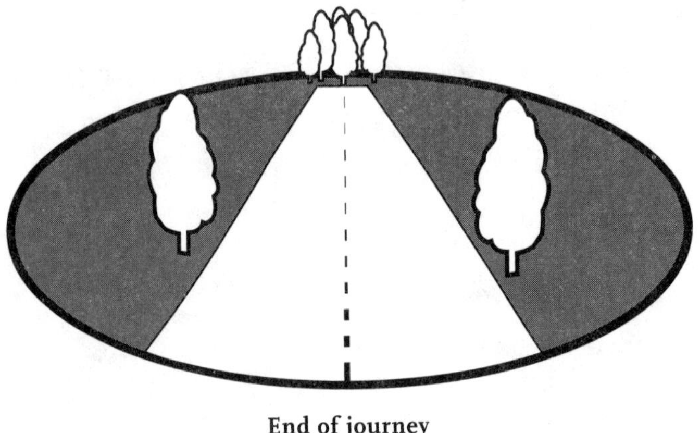

End of journey

Kevin is the last of our "Select Six," an emotional person who represents those who react strongly to the cardiac event. In this chapter, he completes the journey of recovery. But we must remember that the journey is only a metaphor; in reality, what you go through does not end at a specific point. It is, rather, a state of body and mind, a dynamic that continues to respond to the stresses and strains of daily life. At this juncture, patients will be returning to the reality of their particular circumstances. If the recovery process has been valuable, then *change* will have occurred—and productive change at that. But this change occurs in the context of our original selves. Kevin cannot help but still be himself! But he has also made gains during this past year, and he will take these gains with him into the future. There are pros and cons to being emotionally sensitive, particularly if a stressful life event occurs. We will raise this with Kevin and his wife in our final forum, at the end of this chapter. We do not expect readers to be exactly like Kevin, but if there are aspects of him that you can identify with, then we will have done our duty. In the same way, if you identify with any of our "Select Six," we ask you to read "Six Journeys," in Part Two, to find out how Tony's obliviousness, Anna's recurrent symptoms, Joe's mood state, Rose's slow recovery and Mary's "busyness" have affected their recoveries.

HOME AT LAST

THE JOURNEY HAS ENDED. For some, it has been very bumpy; others have taken it in stride. No one was unimpressed: the event had a strong impact on all. We will go over why we need to keep this impression in place. We'll start off by discussing whether one can, in fact, recover from CAD. The event and experience of CAD can be recovered from, but, while CAD *per se* is thought by some to be "reversible," this is not a straightforward notion. We'll then explain what we mean by "recovery," reiterating what will have been achieved both medically and emotionally. We'll then discuss what still has to be done in an ongoing way, and pause to emphasize the challenge of maintenance and remind readers that it is difficult in the long term to successfully maintain the modification of risk factors. We'll explain how to approach this important challenge of maintaining heart-healthy habits, then conclude with a forum on recovery.

CAN I RECOVER FROM CAD?

SOME PEOPLE MAY raise their eyebrows when reading about "recovery" in relation to CAD. We want to make some distinctions between the "event" of CAD, such as heart attack or bypass surgery; the "experience" of CAD, which comprises what we have been describing in this book; and, finally, CAD "itself."

In terms of the *event*, there will be a new equilibrium in the function of the heart following the blockage of the coronary arteries. While the process of *emotional recovery* takes its time, we have witnessed how, in spite of periodic slips, there is usually a new balance arrived at. We have outlined a series of phases or stages through which the patient passes. Labeling the phases of the journey is an artificial thing, and overlap occurs, especially between recuperation and rehabilitation, but by seeing the journey of recovery as a stepwise process we are better able to understand what we are going through. The process of emotional recovery starts with an initial freeze, then a thaw, often followed by a vulnerable emotional reaction. Once reconstruction in the rehabilitation phase takes effect, forward movement is much more assured, until the balance within and between body and mind, and with significant others, is restored. Sustaining the new balance will make for a good recovery.

Most cardiologists feel that one cannot recover completely from CAD *per se*, as one can, for example, from pneumonia or a broken leg. Until recently, it was felt that all one could do was slow the advancement of CAD. There is now some evidence that the narrowing of the coronary arteries can not only be slowed down, but, possibly, actually reversed. This is derived from a few, relatively small studies that showed a slight but significant reopening of the coronary arteries. In these studies, a rigorous treatment routine of very low fat intake, regular exercise and stress management, including group sessions, was established. It is still too early to declare these findings definitive, but they are hopeful. As it is difficult for people to adhere to these programs on an ongoing basis, it would be important if the same effect could be achieved with a less rigorous program.

WHAT IS *REALISTIC* RECOVERY?

Before dealing with recovery itself, you must be reminded about the "art of the possible," not the impossible. In this case, we are going to have to climb down from the pulpit of generalization to ask you what you know about your *own* cardiac event and how you have physically recovered from it. Since every patient is different, every program will be a little different. From a physical standpoint, what has your physician told you about what happened and how you have done until now? Rose cannot expect to feel as well or be as active as the other five patients we have met in this book. Just because Anna has had a very bumpy ride, one cannot be sure that her now-stabilized condition is necessarily worse than those of the others. Since all of you who have an ongoing condition (CAD) are left with the consequences of the cardiac event, you need to maintain yourselves physically, as much as possible. More of that in a moment.

Your body will be affected if you overdo things. You will need to be medically monitored at regular intervals, and continue your ongoing treatments, which usually include medication. Medications that can prevent cardiac deterioration or further events are effective only as long as patients keep using them. In other words, these are lifelong therapies and represent control, not cure. These comments also apply to the emotional side, which is inextricably linked to a physical recovery. Overzealous expectations will lead to inevitable disappointment; being realistic is a sensible and centering attitude.

From the emotional recovery standpoint, "recovery" means having mostly completed a process. A new balance has been achieved and is sustained. Not only are there changes in attitudes and habits, but the patient has come to terms with the new self that has emerged on the journey. As Figure 7.1 shows, the circle is now

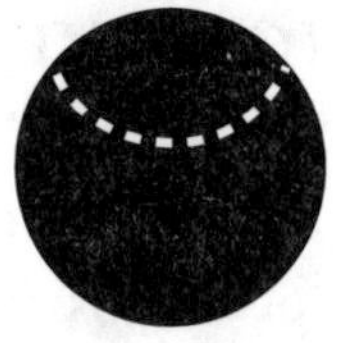

Fig. 7.1
Circle complete—
Recovery

complete. The tint is homogeneous, and the border strongly defined. This represents the establishment of the new self—the boundaries are as solid as the substance within. However, the hatched lines represent what is left of the impact of the event. It is important that *evidence* of an impact *remains*, otherwise you may become careless enough to put yourself at risk again, something that you would not want to do and which would be an example of maladaptive, not adaptive, denial. Recovered individuals will have incorporated the gains made from the other phases, especially those of empowerment. These are flexible strengths that can be used for other eventualities. A key point is for you to be aware of, and be prepared for, symptoms and events that may occur (see "Slippage," pages 112–113). When we stated above that the recovery process was "mostly completed," we were making an important point. You never quite complete the process; you are in a state of ongoing renewal, to maintain your heart-healthy lifestyle and remain under your doctor's management for CAD.

Besides, there are always advantages to a journey you didn't willingly set out on, including something that you *learned* from the crisis. We are sure that you have learned *something* from this book! You should know that the Chinese word for "crisis" means "dangerous opportunity." This event has given you the opportunity to learn new methods and develop your own abilities and strengths for other journeys of your life.

WHAT DO I STILL NEED TO DO?

BY THIS STAGE YOU should be more comfortable with the new routine of your changed habits, which will include an increased commitment to regular activities and exercise, and careful attention to your diet. You will also be accustomed to taking your medication regularly and faithfully. Most rehabilitation programs reduce the need for attendance over time, but occasionally contact with your program can be very useful and rewarding. You can even set an example to those just starting out on their journey (see Joe).

You have come a long way since the original event, and much has changed since you were first hospitalized with heart disease. Although the journey through the aftermath, recuperation and rehabilitation has been a long and difficult one, we hope that you now understand how you came to be where you are and are now much better. Unlike other journeys, this one never really ends. *Staying* well is similar to, but in some respects different from, *getting* well. You will have by now learned more about your heart, and we hope you have adopted healthier heart habits than you had previously. For those of you who had no risk factors for heart disease prior to your event, we hope that you have nevertheless proceeded with rehabilitation and are now aware of those habits you need to maintain to minimize your risk of recurrence.

The most difficult part of any change is wanting to change. Actually making the changes necessary to protect your heart can be difficult, but staying "changed" is not quite as difficult. If you have engaged in a formal exercise rehabilitation program, you will likely now be in the maintenance phase, which is less intensive but still requires ongoing and regular participation in some form of exercise. As the drama of the original illness fades into memory, it is tempting to "coast" and slip back into former ways of living and thinking. Remember that it takes many decades for hardening of the arteries to develop, and that a few months of rigorous adherence to heart-healthy habits cannot reverse a process that may have begun in your twenties or thirties.

The good news is that reducing your risk factors and receiving the best possible medical care after a heart attack is a benefit that continues to grow over the years, and that however advanced your heart disease may be, it is never too late to intervene in a positive way to reduce the chances of another heart attack or other heart problems. In technical terms, death rates after a heart attack in patients receiving treatments known to be beneficial, such as cholesterol-lowering drugs, beta-blocker therapy, and/or exercise rehabilitation, continue to be different from those for patients not so treated; this indicates ongoing and continued benefit from the treatment over time. The flip side, of course, is that the treatment must be continued indefinitely for it to continue to work effectively. Resuming smoking, for example, or stopping your heart medications, or gradually slipping back into a high-fat, fast-food diet, will carry you back where you started in short order.

Patients find that the easiest way to stay on the right road is to focus on the positive achievements they have made during recovery and rehabilitation. For most, this will include a greater sense of control and mastery over their illness, a clear understanding of why they need to follow medical advice, and what the various medications are for.

Research studies have isolated certain beliefs that encourage patients to stick to their therapy. These include a belief that the condition for which treatment is prescribed is a potentially serious one; a belief that the treatment being offered or made available is effective; a belief that they are able to follow the treatment; and a belief that, when they follow the treatment carefully, their quality of life will be better. For most patients, these factors clearly apply.

Most importantly, we hope that this book has helped change your understanding of the way your "biological destiny" and your mind interact. Changing long-standing habits is difficult, and motivating oneself to get started and maintain a personal program is a challenge. Merely knowing that carrot sticks are healthier than chocolate-chip cookies won't decrease the appeal of the cookies! Working on the right frame of mind, however, has double benefits. First, a consistent and thorough commitment to protecting your heart has obvious benefits in reducing the risk of potentially fatal future events. In addition, learning and practicing an attitude of committed, realistic optimism will likely have benefits over and above helping you adopt habits of healthy-heart living. Optimism instead of pessimism, acceptance rather than denial, reaching out instead of letting go, are habits of mind that, in and of themselves, appear to help heart patients feel better and perhaps live longer.

THE CHALLENGE OF MAINTENANCE

THE PROBLEM WITH maintenance is that, in the long term, it is *very difficult to sustain.* Most people we meet have not been able to keep up with moderate low-fat nutrition, never mind a very low-fat diet. The same applies to exercise. How can you overcome this? Are we, as doctors, convinced that it benefits our patients to continue these practices? Of course we are!

Two things prevent you from achieving a new lifestyle: First, your previous habits were ingrained. Second, they were nice! They were enjoyable! Why should you deny yourself this? Because so much of what is *not* allowed is also nice and enjoyable. However, your pleasure centers may be spoiled. You need to persuade them, and there is only one way to do it: *by replacing old, unhealthy habits with new habits that are pleasurable!* You must do things that you *want* to do. It is as simple as that. If, at the recovery stage, you are doing exercise that you don't like, stop!—but find alternatives that you *do* like. There is such a wide choice that everybody can find *some* activity they like to do. Once you have done it once, repeat it. Make sure that your pleasure center is aware of this, because once it is, you don't have to do anything; it will "want" to do it! The same applies to eating. Start the ball rolling with foods that you enjoy. If you are tempted by unhealthy foods, remove them from your home! This is not easy to do with others, such as children, in the house, but a compromise can be reached. To repeat, *you need to develop pleasurable heart-healthy habits.*

FAMILY NOTE

IN ORDER FOR the patient to remain healthy, it is important for the spouse to be part of the recovery process, by keeping family life in balance and being aware when things are off-kilter. The spouse must watch for these things, including a change for the worse in the patient's health. The most predictable slippage will be in risk-factor modification, such as smoking, and lapses in diet and exercise, and you can do the patient and your family a service by helping to meet this challenge. You need also be aware, not only of slippage, but of recurrence, or even an emergency. By now, you will know what you can do to expedite help and treatment as efficiently as possible. Lastly, though more emphasis has been placed on the patient during his or her journey, particularly during the early phases, there comes a time in your relationship for a "completion of the circle," a return to normal, for making the preservation of your own self a priority. You and the patient will both benefit from your seeing yourselves as complete human beings, secure in your self-esteem, who can look forward to other journeys together in the future.

KEEPING A BALANCE

WE HIGHLIGHTED THE importance of seeking a *new* balance in your life. This includes your physical health, your emotional well-being and your social support system. Life is an interacting dynamic, and you need to ensure that you don't go off balance, and, if you do, that you don't remain there. You will want to ensure that your marriage and your family are not in states of persistent unhappiness or conflict, and you are not emotionally distanced from your loved ones. You will want to avoid job strain, heavy financial pressure and estrangement from your family, friends and activities.

How do you do this? On the positive side, your happiness will be linked to a sense of harmony and balance, within yourself and in relation to others. On the cardiac side, by now you "know" what you have to do. Risk-factor modification is an ongoing lifestyle issue and will be much easier to maintain if your emotional life is in balance.

Ten steps to equanimity

One dictionary definition of "equanimity" is "evenness of mind or temper; composure." This represents an attitude of balance between reacting to, or denial of, what has happened up to now, and the unrealistic expectation that heart disease will have no impact on your future well-being or future prospects. Equanimity emphasizes a balance that includes attention paid to your physical, social, emotional and spiritual self. Much as exercise programs continue indefinitely, this process of increasing self-awareness should continue indefinitely. Better understanding of how and why you react to your illness, your loved ones and the stresses and strains in your life will help you be better able to deal with these and continue with the gains that you have made during your rehabilitation.

1. **Listen to your body.** If during an activity you feel physically distressed, it is probably unwise for you to be doing it. This does not mean that a small amount of fatigue, or even shortness of breath, is dangerous and can't, in fact, be energizing. Learn to take the "temperature" of your physical sensations; working somewhat harder at physical activity and being slightly tired is not dangerous and can be a sign that you are getting physical training. Learn also to distinguish true physical hunger from feeling like eating something that you may not need nutritionally. Try to distinguish "I want" from "I need," and "I can't" from "I won't."

2. **Listen to your loved ones.** Most of us are fortunate to have significant others, family members or trusted friends who have our welfare at heart and are able to be more objective about our condition than we ourselves can be. Listening carefully to their advice, even if we don't always heed it precisely, can help us feel that we are part of a team rather than "going it alone."

3. **Seek professional advice.** This includes from your doctors, staff at a cardiac rehabilitation clinic, a nutritionist, physiotherapist, spiritual adviser, and anyone you may have access to who can help you with specific aspects of your rehabilitation. Remember, they have your best interests in mind.

4. **Be contemplative.** Think carefully about the journey you are on, where you have come from and where you are heading, and what you need to do to stay on the right road. This includes

appropriate use of hesitation. If you are about to turn the TV on, thinking, "Oh, I'm too tired to take a walk tonight," consider whether this is what you really would like to do. Which activity will make you feel better about yourself, and ultimately give you more life satisfaction? Before you reach for that second piece of chocolate cake, hesitate; think of the positive benefits of taking control over your eating habits, which will make it easier for you to hesitate the next time.

5. **Understand and follow your medical regimen.** Fortunately, there are many effective and life-prolonging medications available to heart patients today. You may need to take many of these. Although you may think that they are a nuisance to take, have annoying side effects and represent a financial commitment, they also have undoubted long-term benefits. Understanding the nature of and the purpose for each of your medications will make it much easier for you to follow the regimen you are prescribed.

6. **Be patient.** Successful rehabilitation and recovery is a slow and ongoing process, and you should not expect to be able to change all of your habits overnight.

7. **Be optimistic.** This may not be an easy frame of mind to adopt, especially when you have been ill. Remember that most patients can achieve remarkable gains in their well-being and capacity for activity if they take it slowly, expect only small changes from day to day, and have faith in the ability of their bodies to improve. Remember, this improvement can take place even if the heart muscle does not itself get stronger, and despite the presence of fairly serious heart disease.

8. **Be realistic.** Set yourself achievable goals. If, for example, you wish to lose weight, don't expect to achieve the entire goal within the next weeks or months. Rather, take it "one pound at a time." If you want to enlarge your circle of friends or your social activities, consider joining one club or one activity at first, and make regular attendance at their meetings or activities a goal.

9. **You're stronger than you think.** Most of us have reserves of untapped energy that we never use, and our bodies are more resilient than we imagine. For example, the *ejection fraction* is the percentage of blood in the heart that is pumped with each beat. Normally this is over 50 percent, or even over 60 percent. Many patients with ejection fractions of 20 or 30 percent, formerly thought to be incapable of any level of exertion, can over time learn to perform almost all the activities of daily life, including the moderately strenuous ones. Over time, patients can completely change their eating habits, and even their outlook on life. Although difficult, change is possible.

10. **The journey is never over.** Remember, you are never truly "cured" of heart disease, but you can learn to live in stable equilibrium with your heart, and if you treat it with respect, it will be less likely to treat you rudely in the future.

FORUM (KEVIN): Looking back and looking forward

Kevin is a forty-six-year-old worker in an automotive plant who was well and had no family history or other risk factors of heart disease. He didn't exercise much, but had a normal weight. While on vacation at a beach resort, he developed chest pain, which he thought was indigestion, and didn't see a doctor about it. After his return home, he had several more of these pains, which were lasting up to an hour, and eventually he went to the hospital to get some antacid medication. He was astounded when the doctors did an electrocardiogram and told him that he was in danger of having a heart attack and had to be hospitalized immediately. The next day he had a coronary angiogram which showed a severe blockage of several arteries, and an urgent bypass was recommended. A week later he had the bypass, from which he physically recovered uneventfully, and at exercise testing six weeks later was able to run on the treadmill without any problems.

At first Kevin was stunned by what had happened, and particularly so when he came home and his wife was very protective toward him. They were counseled by their family doctor, and his wife responded to this, but for some time Kevin felt anxious about what had happened and was still worried about having a heart attack. When his fears subsided, he was troubled by feelings of anger about the unfairness of this having happened to him. Later, once he became involved in the rehab program, he calmed considerably and started to feel much better.

This forum consists of Kevin, his wife, Dr Dorian and Dr Baker.

KEVIN: Well, doctor, how do you think I've done?

DR DORIAN: How do *you* think you have done?

KEVIN: At first it was quite a roller coaster, but now that seems in the past. You know the whole story. My wife especially took it real hard. Isn't that so, dear?

WIFE: You can say that again. I couldn't stop crying when I heard that he had to have the surgery, and later, when he came home, I wouldn't let him out of my sight.

KEVIN: Yes, that got on my nerves.

WIFE: You can't blame me for being upset about that. It was so out of the blue. One moment, we're on vacation at the beach; a few days later, they're operating on your heart! At first, I couldn't stop checking on him, but once we spoke to our doctor I felt I could handle things. Kevin took longer than me to calm down.

KEVIN: Well, it is *my* heart!

DR BAKER: Usually the patient is emotionally upset for longer than the spouse.

KEVIN: Now I'm feeling well, but sometimes I wonder if it's better that I know all about my heart disease; then it seems like such a load to carry around with me. Maybe I would have been better off if I would have been one of those guys who didn't give a hoot about things. Don't they say "ignorance is bliss"?

WIFE: Kevin's just joking. Once he understood what had happened to him, he started to accept his condition.

DR DORIAN: After some initial bumps in the road, you have come to understand that heart disease is part of you, and this is unfortunately a disease for life that will not disappear. At the same time, you now know that the disease can be managed and that with knowledge about your heart and your body come understanding, and with understanding comes the chance for serenity. Some other patients never get over their angry phase, and cannot concentrate enough to learn the value of modifying their habits or complying with their treatment regimen.

KEVIN: But I was perfectly well until this all happened.

DR DORIAN: Many of our patients suffer a cardiac event without any prior warning whatsoever, and indeed have no risk factors. They ask, "How could this happen to me? I have done all the right things, watched my diet, I don't smoke, I exercise and still my arteries are my enemy." We believe that in many of these patients, arterial narrowing is caused by factors that they have no control over, such as a genetic predisposition (even though they may not have family members affected), possibly subtle biochemical abnormalities in their blood, or even infections that can predispose to arterial narrowing. It's very important that patients understand that in most cases it is not their fault that they have developed artery disease, and that it is not right or useful for patients to be angry at themselves or for family members to be angry at patients for having developed this disease.

KEVIN: Do you think that things were worse for me because they came on so suddenly?

DR BAKER: Yes, the suddenness does add an extra edge to things, but we also have to deal with how you handle stress generally.

WIFE: There are still times when I worry about Kevin.

Dr Baker: Why?

Wife: Well, he still can still get upset easily, and if there is something bothering him, he won't let it go.

Dr Baker: Each person has to deal with his or her own character and temperament. Frankly, after many years of trying to change people, I have learned that the trick is to know what you cannot change! If you are aware of that large component, then you can deal with what you *are* able to change. Kevin will probably continue to get upset in certain situations, but hopefully, since he is now aware of what upsets him, and knows some techniques to deal with it better, it won't be so often, or so strong, or go on for as long as before.

Kevin: Like I said, I've come to terms with the fact that I will always have some heart trouble, but I have stopped blaming myself and everyone else for the fact that I have heart disease, and I am no longer so upset or angry with myself when I do fly off the handle, since I know that no one can be on a perfectly even keel all the time. The doctors have also told me not to be so worried that every time I get upset it will affect my heart and cause another heart attack.

Wife: It's true that you are much better, but you sound as if you have everything under control. I notice you aren't exercising as often as before, and at times we do cheat on the diet.

Kevin: As a matter of fact, I am still walking three times a week, and don't forget I do quite a lot of exercise at work. My wife is only talking about when we go out to eat once a week. Anyway, my cholesterol is normal.

Dr Dorian: As long as you generally follow the dietary recommendations, and especially if your blood tests are okay, occasional "cheating" is not a problem.

Wife: If I think back, it was when he became active that he really started to turn around.

Kevin: Yes, it was when I went to the rehab program. Once I got started with the exercise, I was supervised and I learned all about my condition; this gave me confidence. Also, when I was back to work with my buddies, all those months of worrying just faded away. It's funny, though, when we talk about it my mind starts to think of all these things again.

Dr Baker: I think there is a time for talking and a time for doing.

Kevin: That's true. You know, I did a lot of talking over the past year, and I learned a lot too. Now I'm ready for other things.

Dr Baker: This is a good point. At this time, we have to strike the right balance between shutting things out of our minds and getting on with our lives, on the one hand, and maintaining a heart-healthy lifestyle, on the other.

Dr Dorian: It is true that living with heart disease is much like being in a relationship. Even when you think you have "got it right," the job is never completely finished. It is this continual working at it that, although it may seem difficult at first, allows you the sense of mastery over your illness that can help you so much in dealing with the inevitable ups and downs.

KEVIN: Well, we know all about being in a relationship. At times it is tough, but it is worth it!

WIFE: You can say that again.

EPILOGUE

Not fare well,
But fare forward, voyagers
—T.S. Eliot

THE END OF a journey is the start of a new one. Life is not just heart disease! While coronary heart disease is part of what we have to carry along on the journey, it is quite compatible with a good quality of life. We will want to take new roads and expand our experience of life. We have incorporated what we have gone through since our cardiac event, but we are not defined only by this experience. This is only a part of the total living of our lives. There are other journeys to travel, and other metaphors to use! So, let us move on.

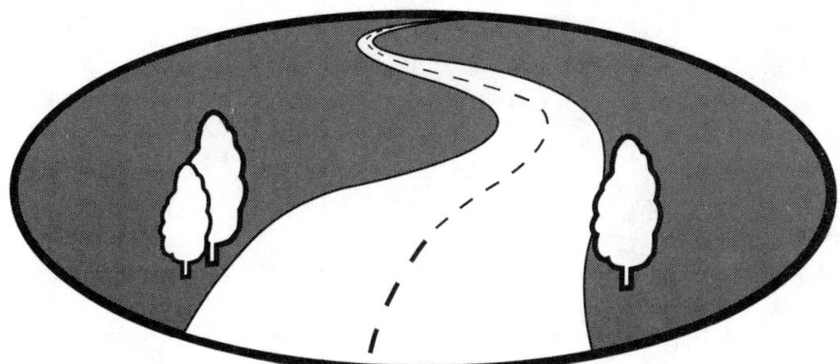

End of journey—start of new one

PART TWO:

Directions

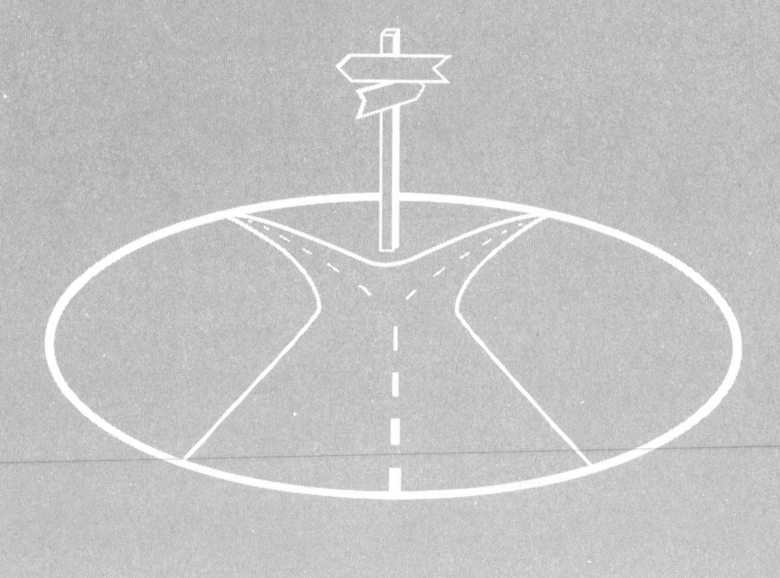

CHAPTER 8

What You Need to Know about "Directions": An Introduction

Part Two, "Directions," is for those who want more "direction," more guidelines or more information. You do not have to read everything here, but whatever interests you, whatever you feel you would like to know, can be found in these pages. There are four chapters in this part: "Heart," "Mind," "Heart to Mind" and "Six Journeys." The first two contain guidelines, or information, for those with CAD and their families. The range of subjects covered is not necessarily complete; rather, it is our personal choice of what you may want to access. We have selected information that we feel incorporates "the basics." For some subjects, we have purposely avoided providing too much detail. For example, in our discussion of clinical depression and cholesterol our goal is simply to alert you to when it becomes necessary to consult a professional, and *not* to substitute for this type of evaluation. In our discussion of rehab programs, we have included basic information and leave the details to the available literature on the subject.

Chapter 9, "Heart: Key Physical Issues for Those with Heart Disease," starts with an overview of CAD, something that many will want to know more about, and explains what happens when you go to the hospital.

It will be invaluable for each person to review what to do in an emergency; the material on tests, procedures and medications will be of interest less generally, based on each person's experience. Again, our reviews should be seen as an introduction and are not to take the place of actual consultation with your doctors.

A practical issue in your treatment is who treats you, so we have included an introduction to your team of professionals. Many readers will be treated in hospitals where valuable medical research on CAD is being conducted, and you may be approached about this.

We open discussion of the important area of prevention with the question, Can you prevent heart disease? We then discuss each risk factor for coronary heart disease, including family history, diabetes, high blood pressure, smoking, sedentary lifestyle, being overweight and cholesterol. We end by highlighting an area, neglected in the past, but fortunately now coming under the spotlight: women and heart disease.

A particular focus of this book is the emphasis on the *experience* of CAD, including the feelings you may experience. This is the subject of Chapter 10, "Mind: Key Emotional Issues for Those with Heart Disease." Anxiety is a common response to the cardiac event, but can persist or have special characteristics, such as panic or fear. For cardiac patients there is the danger of an overlap with physical symptoms, causing a vicious circle. Depression is also common after a cardiac event, but we will need to distinguish the normal response of low mood from clinical depression and persistent low mood, which require consultation and treatment. The emotional aspect can be quite confusing to many and for this reason we have included a section on when to seek counseling, and from whom.

We tackle the thorny question of whether stress can cause coronary heart disease by explaining that the relation is a complex one, with stress acting as a trigger rather than a cause. Certain stressors have been isolated, and we review them and the stress-management techniques designed to deal with them. The key components of stress management which are most frequently emphasized are relaxation techniques, and time and anger management, including assertiveness training. We mention the problem of the sensitive person and focus on a recurring finding that social isolation is not good for your cardiac health. In the mind of the patient there is often no doubt about the link between stress and CAD. In a patient's personal perspective, we report verbatim a "from the heart" account written by one of our patients. We conclude with a mention of two possible psychiatric emergencies—acute depression and panic attacks.

Although we have tried to speak "with one voice," at times it is useful to disclose the origins of the separate voices, which represent the different specialties of cardiology and psychiatry. In Chapter 11, "Heart to Mind," we give three dialogues on key areas in the journey of recovery. The first, "The third way," develops the notion of how the interaction of the specialties can add to our understanding of the response to the cardiac event. "Themes of healing" explores the important area of recuperation, which at first is a time of contrast between the body and mind. The final discussion revolves around a crucial question at the cusp of the upbeat phase of rehabilitation—when are you "ready for rehabilitation"? Readers may find the information here somewhat technical, because we are talking as specialists to each other, but we still want you to eavesdrop.

Finally, there are always readers who prefer to read about what actually happened. They want to know the stories. Case histories are able to specify what can happen to particular patients. In Chapter 12, "Six Journeys," we tell the stories of our "Select Six" cardiac patients. These stories emphasize the emotional side, reflecting our focus in this book: the experience of heart disease. Tony represents those who turn a blind eye to their treatment; Anna is someone who has experienced repeated episodes (cardiac events); Rose illustrates what happens when you don't get back to normal. Mary is someone whose life is activity-based. Joe is stalled. Kevin is the one leaning most to the emotional side of the spectrum. Each story has "layers" that unfold as you go along. (The backgrounds to these stories are provided in Part One, "The Guide.")

CHAPTER 9

Heart: Key Physical Issues for Those with Heart Disease

WHAT IS HEART DISEASE?

HEART DISEASE IS any problem or disorder of the *heart*, which is simply and basically a pump that receives "blue" blood, which has little oxygen, from the body, and whose right side pumps it to the lungs. "Red" blood, rich in oxygen, is then returned to the left side of the heart and pumped to the body by the main, strongest heart chamber, the *left ventricle*.

As is true of any other part of the body, many diseases can affect the heart. These include (but are not limited to) problems with the heart valves, problems with the arteries (the "plumbing") and infections of the heart. The most important and by far the most common of heart diseases (in the Western world) are caused by *hardening of the arteries*, causing narrowing or blockage of the arteries that supply the heart muscle itself with blood and oxygen. This process, called *atherosclerosis*, can begin at a young or middle age, although most patients don't begin to have problems until their sixth, seventh or later decades of life.

What happens when you get hardening of the arteries?

The arteries harden when deposits containing cholesterol and scar tissue ("plaque") build up inside them and gradually choke off the blood supply. This prevents the heart muscle from getting enough blood and oxygen to pump effectively. Lack of oxygen, most often occurring during the exertion of exercise or mental stress, can cause pain known as *angina*. This is usually perceived as chest tightness, heaviness or squeezing discomfort, sometimes also felt in the neck, jaws, left arm or back. The discomfort usually subsides after a few minutes' rest.

How does a heart attack happen?

When the plaque or fatty deposit in the artery wall is irritated or injured, a clot can form inside the artery and this may block off blood flow altogether. If blood supply is completely interrupted for long enough, a *heart attack* ensues. A heart attack invariably causes some amount of heart damage—in other words, the death of heart muscle cells that are then replaced by scar tissue.

Why is a heart attack risky?

In the hours to days following a heart attack, there is a risk of serious heart rhythm disturbances ("electrical disturbances"), and severe weakness of the heart muscle as a pump. After initial recovery, a number of late problems can occur: the heart muscle can continue to be weak, and be unable to pump enough blood to meet the body's needs. This can result in fatigue, weakness and shortness of breath from what is known as "heart failure," which results in a higher pressure than normal in the lungs, causing shortness of breath. This shortness of breath most often occurs with activity, or at nighttime.

Sometimes the heart attack is incomplete, and chest pain or tightness can return, technically known as *post-infarction angina.* Heart rhythm disturbances can also occur, causing a rapid heart rhythm known as *ventricular tachycardia*, which is caused by a short circuit close to the scar of the heart attack. These short circuits, if they are present, can become activated for no obvious reason and cause a very rapid heartbeat which leads to dizziness, severe light-headedness or loss of consciousness that can be life-threatening or even cause death, although fortunately this is not common. A less serious but troublesome heart rhythm disturbance is *atrial fibrillation*, an irregular heart rhythm that causes palpitations and dizziness but is rarely life threatening.

Complications of coronary heart disease or associated conditions

The four major categories of illness produced by or associated with coronary heart disease are clots forming inside blood vessels or the heart, known as *thrombosis*; *myocardial ischemia and infarction* (heart attack); weakness of the heart muscle leading to *heart failure*; and rhythm disturbances of the heart, also known as *arrhythmia.*

Thrombosis, or clot formation, can cause stroke if the blockage is in the arteries (blood vessels) in the brain, or in the neck (where large blood vessels that supply brain blood flow are located), with the clots "flowing" away to the brain vessels. Sometimes clots form and dissolve, causing a temporary interruption of brain blood flow (leading to temporary blindness, double vision, numbness or paralysis, difficulty with speech or understanding speech, dizziness or loss of balance, sometimes associated with headache). If fully reversible, these are called *transient ischemic attacks* (*TIAs*), a temporary loss of blood supply to the brain. If the blood flow is permanently cut off, a *stroke* results, which does lead to permanent brain damage. However, there is often very substantial recovery from a stroke as the brain swelling caused by blood-flow interruption subsides and as nondamaged parts of the brain take over some of the functions of the damaged part.

More rarely, clots can travel to other body organs and interrupt their function, including the kidneys, intestines and the legs. Such a clot that travels downstream to plug up a smaller artery is called an *embolus*. These clots occur in the *arteries*, blood vessels that carry "red" blood rich in oxygen away from the heart to various body locations.

Sometimes clots can form in veins (which carry "blue" blood, from which the oxygen has been removed in its passage through various body tissues). Most often these clots form in the veins of the upper legs or pelvis. Such clots are more common in patients with heart disease, especially heart failure. They may travel back to the heart, and through the right side of the heart into the lungs, where they can cause a *pulmonary embolus*, a blood clot in the lung. This can cause shortness of breath, chest pain and a rapid hearbeat, and may lead to collapse. If diagnosed early, such clots can be effectively treated with blood thinners, and rarely clot busters, or even surgery to remove the clot.

The cause of the heart damage in a heart attack and the consequences have been described in Part One. In brief, if blood supply to the heart is completely interrupted for many minutes or longer, the heart muscle cells begin to die. Beyond thirty minutes of no blood flow to a portion of the heart muscle, permanent damage is almost inevitable, although the amount of damage will depend on the size of the blood vessel blocked, on the oxygen needs of the heart muscle that is deprived of nutrition, and on the length of time during which there is no blood supply. The consequences of heart damage or a heart attack are largely related to the heart muscle weakness it causes, which in turn impairs the pumping action of the heart and can cause *heart failure*.

Heart failure is a condition where the heart is sufficiently damaged that it can no longer pump blood effectively to meet the body's needs. Heart failure can result in weakness, fatigue, lack of energy and lightheadedness. When the heart fails to pump enough blood through the body, more blood is left in the heart cavity at the end of each heartbeat. This increased amount of blood exerts pressure on the inner walls of the heart, and this can lead to a "backup of blood" behind the heart (much like water "backs up" behind a dam), accumulating in the lungs. This is known as *congestive heart failure*, during which patients have shortness of breath on exertion, or occasionally even at rest; may find it difficult to lie flat because of shortness of breath; have trouble sleeping because of cough or waking up short of breath; as well as suffering from appetite loss, bloating, and swelling of the feet, ankles and legs. Congestive heart failure is associated with more salt and water in the body than is normal. Patients with this condition need to be very careful about their salt intake, and avoid salty foods, many prepared foods (which are very high in salt) and excessive added salt at the table. They are usually prescribed *diuretics* ("water pills") which help get rid of salt and water through the kidneys, as well as other medications. These are described in detail below.

Arrhythmias are disturbances of the heart's rhythm, which occur commonly in patients with a recent heart attack or coronary artery disease. They can arise from the pumping chambers of the heart known as the *ventricles*, or from the collecting chambers of the heart known as the *atria*. Most *ventricular arrhythmias* usually don't cause patients to suffer. They generally occur as premature or "extra" beats, which are often not felt by patients, or perceived as "skipped beats" or a momentary sensation of a "hollow feeling" in the chest or a "pause" in the heartbeat, followed by a single forceful or prominent heartbeat. Such extra beats are not in and of themselves dangerous, but may indicate that the individual is more likely than others to develop serious forms of heart rhythm disturbance. These serious forms include *ventricular tachycardia* and *ventricular fibrillation. Ventricular tachycardia* is a rapid, regular heartbeat that is caused by a "short circuit" arising in the vicinity of a scar from a previous heart attack. This short circuit may be present early or develop very late after a heart attack, but once it forms it does not generally disappear. For mysterious reasons, such short circuits are "activated," i.e., "switched on," only occasionally and intermittently, and, when they are, the patient suddenly develops a rapid heartbeat with palpitations, dizziness, or even loss of consciousness. If not treated promptly, ventricular tachycardia can be dangerous, or even fatal. The most effective treatment is an electrical shock to the heart through paddles on the chest wall, known as *cardioversion*. Such shocks are usually delivered by paramedics, ambulance personnel, or doctors in emergency rooms or coronary care units; fortunately, these days, this life-saving treatment may also be available from other individuals such as firemen, policemen and other trained persons in the community who have access to the very useful devices known as *defibrillators*, machines that can deliver shocks to restore a normal heartbeat. Such devices may be manually operated or may be automatic—in other words, decide on their own if a shock is required, with the operator merely needed to push a button to allow the machine to work independently. It is not known why *ventricular tachycardia* arises when it does, and usually there is no particular explanation at the time of the particular event. Although it is commonly believed that mental, emotional or physical stress can cause these rhythm disturbances, there is no clear proof that there is any precipitant that is consistently the culprit.

A more severe form of heart rhythm disturbance is *ventricular fibrillation*, a very rapid and completely disorganized and irregular beating of the pumping chambers (ventricles), which invariably leads to collapse and death within a few minutes unless cardiopulmonary resuscitation (CPR) and defibrillation are promptly available and used. Ventricular fibrillation is the most common cause of *cardiac arrest*, a condition where there is no effective heart pumping. Unfortunately, the single most common serious complication after heart attack is such rhythm disturbances, which can occur quite unpredictably and without warning.

How are serious arrhythmias treated?

If a person develops a life-threatening heart rhythm such as ventricular fibrillation, there is no effective blood flow to the brain and vital organs, and without treatment death will ensue within ten to fifteen minutes. Some degree of blood flow can be restored by *cardiopulmonary resuscitation* (*CPR*), which involves mouth-to-mouth breathing and chest compressions and is now widely taught under the auspices of organizations such as the Heart and Stroke Foundation of Canada and its affiliates, in hospitals and in universities, and has become a part of first-aid instruction. Perhaps the most important component of CPR is the ability to recognize a serious cardiac emergency such as *cardiac arrest.* Such patients will not respond when spoken to or shaken, will not be breathing or will be making shallow and feeble efforts at respiration, and do not have a pulse (which can usually be felt at the wrist or at the neck), but may be moving or having slight convulsive movements. Acting promptly in such an emergency can be truly life saving. The most important first action is to call for professional rescue, in most communities by dialing 911. If CPR is then begun, the period of grace until irreversible brain injury occurs will be prolonged by up to many minutes, thus possibly allowing effective resuscitation if trained paramedics or other trained personnel arrive promptly on the scene.

The only way to restore an effective heartbeat in the case of *ventricular fibrillation* is to deliver an electrical shock to the heart, known as *defibrillation*, using paddles or patches applied to the chest wall. Even if advanced care and defibrillation are available, not all patients with out-of-hospital cardiac arrest will be rescued; even under ideal circumstances, only about 20 to 30 percent of such patients survive in the long term. However, this minority can be restored to a good quality of life, and these patients may, if fortunate enough to survive, have excellent long-term prospects.

Contrary to popular belief, most such cases of sudden cardiac collapse are *not* caused by a "massive heart attack," but by such an "electrical accident" as ventricular fibrillation (usually in a patient with prior heart disease).

What happens if a patient is rescued (resuscitated) from a cardiac arrest?

Without specific treatment, these patients are prone to having another serious event such as another cardiac arrest. Fortunately, there are very effective treatments available. Most of these patients will undergo a variety of cardiac tests, including *electrocardiograms*, an *echocardiogram* (ultrasound), *exercise testing*, and often *cardiac catheterization with an angiogram* (page 162). Many of them will also have a form of electrical testing known as *electrophysiologic study*. The treatment may include drugs to stabilize heart rhythm, or a device known as an *implanted cardioverter defibrillator*, which is a miniature, automatic device the size of a small bar of soap that is implanted in the body and automatically detects and treats a rapid life-threatening heart rhythm if it occurs. Other treatments may include a variety of other drugs, or bypass surgery.

Atrial fibrillation is the most common heart rhythm disturbance. Unlike *ventricular fibrillation*, it is not life-threatening and does not cause collapse, loss of consciousness, heart attack or heart damage. It is, however, extremely common and can moderately or even severely impair quality of life. This rhythm disturbance arises in the collecting chambers of the heart (known as the *atria*), and leads to a rapid, irregular heartbeat that is less efficient than a normal heartbeat. Patients with this rhythm disorder suffer from palpitations, lightheadedness, shortness of breath and weakness in varying degrees of severity. These symptoms can be intermittent or continuous. Atrial fibrillation can be very effectively treated, but requires close follow-up with a physician expert in its care. Many patients with atrial fibrillation will be at risk for clot formation inside the heart, which can lead to stroke. This can be very effectively prevented by a blood thinner called *warfarin*, whose use is detailed below.

What about slow heartbeats?

A completely different type of set of heart rhythm disturbances are those that lead to excessive slowing of the heartbeat (in contrast to rapid heartbeats). These occur relatively commonly in patients with a history of a heart attack. The normal heartbeat is a contraction, or beating, of the pumping chambers of the heart in response to electrical signals that begin in the natural heart pacemaker (the *sinoatrial node*), which is located in the right collecting chamber, or *right atrium.* The electrical signals generated by this natural biologic pacemaker are conducted through the heart's "wiring" to the ventricles or pumping chambers. If the normal heart pacemaker functions improperly, the heartbeat will be excessively slow. Similarly, if the electrical wiring connecting the normal biological pacemaker to the *ventricles* (pumping chambers) is malfunctioning, the heartbeat will also be slow. Such slowing can lead to dizziness, lightheadedness, weakness, or even loss of consciousness. Fortunately, even severe heartbeat slowing is rarely immediately fatal, and is easily treatable. *Pacemakers*, extremely effective for the treatment of *slow* heartbeats, provide electrical signals to the ventricles that stimulate them to contract, resulting in a regular heartbeat at a normal rate. Pacemakers are implanted during a brief operation, which may last only an hour or so, through a small incision under the left or right collarbone, and the pacemaker itself, which is about the size of the body of a wristwatch, is connected to the heart by means of a flexible wire (*lead*) that delivers the electrical impulses to the ventricles. The batteries in these devices last seven to twelve years, and patients can lead entirely normal lives when they have pacemakers. Contrary to what many people think, pacemakers are perfectly safe around various home and industrial appliances, including microwave ovens, refrigerators, airport metal detectors, and so on. Patients with pacemakers face no restrictions whatsoever from their usual activities, including physical exercise.

WHAT TO DO IN AN EMERGENCY

FORTUNATELY, TRUE EMERGENCIES are rarely observed in patients with heart disease, but you must recognize the warning signs if they do happen. The most serious of these emergencies is a sudden severe heart rhythm disturbance called *ventricular tachycardia* or *ventricular fibrillation*, which causes a very rapid and sometimes disorganized heart beating, leading to loss of effective heart pumping. This can cause sudden severe dizziness, or loss of consciousness. If the heart pump is very severely affected, a *cardiac arrest* can occur, during which the heart does not pump blood at all. This is a life-threatening emergency; *CPR* (*cardiopulmonary resuscitation*) needs to be started right away, and an ambulance should be called immediately. For this problem, only advanced care from paramedics or other personnel, usually requiring an electrical shock to the heart (defibrillation), can restore proper heart beating. The important signs are severe dizziness, collapse and loss of consciousness, especially if they last more than a few seconds. Time is of the essence.

Severe shortness of breath, often accompanied by a dry cough and weakness, can mean *acute congestive heart failure*. In this condition, blood backs up "into the lungs" from a poorly beating heart. If a person is severely short of breath at rest, especially if he or she has difficulty lying flat or is coughing severely, an ambulance needs to be called. This condition is treatable, and patients do much better if it is caught early.

Many patients with heart disease will frequently have chest discomfort or tightness that lasts only a few minutes at a time, is brought on by physical or emotional stress and is relieved by rest. Sometimes, these sensations are more severe and do not go away quickly. If chest pain or tightness lasts more than thirty minutes, particularly if it is accompanied by sweating, shortness of breath and weakness, the patient might have unstable angina or a heart attack (*myocardial infarction*). In this case, medical help is needed right away, preferably from a hospital emergency department.

WHAT HAPPENS WHEN YOU GO TO THE HOSPITAL?

IN ANY PATIENT with suspected *coronary artery disease* (hardening of the arteries), the most common reason for seeking urgent medical help is prolonged chest pain, chest tightness, shortness of breath or weakness. These symptoms often result in patients' going to an emergency room, or consulting with their doctors urgently. The two important questions that the doctors ask themselves are: (1) Are the symptoms due to lack of blood supply to the heart (*myocardial ischemia*) or some other medical problem?; and (2) Are you having a heart attack?

The first question is important since the presence of *myocardial ischemia* almost always means that hospitalization is required, often in a *coronary care unit*, and involves intensive medical therapy (detailed below) and close observation, with continuous monitoring of your *electrocardiogram* (*ECG*). It is also crucial for doctors to decide if you are in the throes of a heart attack, since the severity of a heart attack can be markedly reduced by using "clot busters," technically known as *thrombolytic drugs*. In heart attack patients who are treated within the first hours after the onset of chest pain or discomfort, these drugs can markedly reduce the risk of death and limit the amount of heart damage that could occur. Currently, the first test used to decide if you are having a heart attack is a simple *electrocardiogram* (*ECG*), during which small electrodes are placed on your chest, arms and legs, in order to record the tiny electrical signals coming from your heart. The usual sign on the electrocardiogram of an ongoing heart attack is what is called *ST segment elevation*; this indicates that you may benefit from clot-busting drugs (unless there is a reason to withhold them, which can occasionally happen). Clot busters are useful for up to six, or even twelve, hours after a heart attack, although their effectiveness diminishes rapidly after the first few hours from the onset of symptoms.

Occasionally, chest pain or chest discomfort suggests symptoms of *myocardial ischemia* (lack of blood supply to the heart) but the electrocardiogram does not definitively indicate a heart attack. To sort this out, blood will be drawn to be analyzed for *myocardial enzymes*, which are substances found inside heart muscle cells that are not normally present in the blood but are released into the blood if heart damage occurs. These tests can indicate heart damage as soon as a few hours into a heart attack. After you are evaluated in an emergency room, and an electrocardiogram and blood tests are done, you will usually be sent to a *coronary care unit.*

Coronary care units were first developed in Toronto, Ontario, in the 1960s, and allow close monitoring of cardiac patients, intensive nursing care and immediate treatment of any complications that may arise. During these early hours, patients are treated with various medications, such as *heparin*, a blood thinner available intravenously; *nitrates*, drugs that dilate blood vessels and improve blood supply to the heart; and often *beta blockers*, drugs that slow the heartbeat and decrease the amount of work the heart has to do. Aspirin is almost always administered, as it prevents blood *platelets* (small circulating elements in the blood that can stick or clump together and indirectly lead to clotting) from sticking together. During the first few days in the coronary care unit, you will undergo daily electrocardiograms, likely several chest X rays, and receive daily visits from your doctor. You will probably also have an ultrasound of your heart (*echocardiogram*) in the first few days, and if your chest pain recurs or persists you may undergo an *angiogram*, an X ray of the blood vessels that supply blood to the heart. (These tests are described in more detail below.) After one to several days in the coronary care unit, depending on whether you have had a heart attack (*myocardial infarction*) or *unstable angina* (a "threatened heart attack" but where actual heart muscle damage does not occur), you will be transferred to a regular hospital ("ward") unit.

Most patients spend a few days to a week in the hospital following an acute cardiac event, unless complications occur or unless a complex procedure or heart surgery is required. Prior to hospital discharge, many patients undergo some form of *exercise testing* to assess the response of the heart to physical stress. Counseling with respect to long-term changes in diet, activity level, exercise, smoking cessation and other lifestyle changes may occur at this time, or may be deferred until after the early convalescence period is over, generally four to six weeks later.

TESTS OFTEN PERFORMED ON PATIENTS WITH HEART DISEASE

PATIENTS WITH HEART disease may undergo a variety of simple and not-so-simple tests. Their purpose and what patients can expect are detailed below.

Cardiac catheterization and coronary angiography: "Cardiac catheterization" is a general term that refers to the placement of tubes inside blood vessels going to the heart, in order to study the heart function. "Coronary angiography" means that a dye is injected into the arteries that supply the heart with blood, and X-ray pictures are taken of these arteries when they are filled with dye. This test produces the most accurate image of the blood vessels that are prone to hardening or narrowing, and allows fairly precise identification of the extent, location, pattern and severity of narrowings or blockages in the blood vessels to the heart. After local anesthetic is injected into the groin area or the arm, a *cardiac catheter*, a long flexible tube, is inserted into the artery and threaded into the heart's chambers, usually the left and sometimes the right *ventricle*. The pressure in this chamber is measured, and then a small amount of dye is injected, after which the *cine angiogram*, or "movie camera," is turned on for a few seconds, to record the image of the dye, which is not transparent to the X-ray beam, as it is ejected from the heart. This is necessary since the heart muscle and the blood are transparent to the X-ray beam and thus the heart is normally invisible with ordinary X rays and the naked eye. This *left ventricular angiogram* gives an accurate image of the strength of pumping action of the heart and of *valvular regurgitation*, or "leaky valves," if present. The catheters are then exchanged for other catheters, which are specially shaped to allow injection of dye directly into the *coronary arteries*, which are the arteries that supply the heart muscle itself and are branches of the aorta (the largest blood vessel in the body, which leads from the heart to the rest of the body. Dye is then injected into the left and the right coronary arteries (the two main trunks from which branches lead), and several different images are taken of each artery, each time after injecting a small amount of dye, and moving the camera so that the arteries may be viewed from several different angles. These images are also stored on film or on computer disk, and can be later reviewed to see the presence and exact appearance of narrowings or blockages. Decisions about the technical suitability of the patient for *angioplasty* or *bypass surgery* are made on the basis of these images.

The entire procedure usually takes about forty-five minutes, and generally is associated with some mild discomfort in the groin area but is not terribly painful. The most unpleasant part of the procedure is the requirement to lie flat on a hard X-ray table; the need to lie still, which can result in some back stiffness; and the understandable anxiety that goes along with having a procedure in an unfamiliar and rather forbidding environment.

Patients are asked to lie flat for four to six hours following the procedure, and are generally up and around and may be discharged either the same day or the next day. Complications of angiograms are relatively rare, the most common being bleeding or bruising where the tubes are inserted. More serious complications such as clot formation in the blood vessels, a heart attack or a stroke are very rare, far less than 1 in 100, usually about 1 in 500. The risk of death from this procedure is extremely small, less than 1 in 1,000.

Echocardiogram (ultrasound): An echocardiogram is much like a "radar" of the heart, and provides an image of the heart using high-frequency sound beams (which cannot be heard) emitted from a probe placed on the chest wall. These sound beams travel through the skin to the heart and bounce back to a detector that allows an image of the heart to be displayed on a TV screen. This is a very accurate test, which can allow measurement of the strength of the heart's beating, the size of the heart and its chambers, localized weakness of the muscles in the heart, problems with the heart valves, and any other structural problem with the heart. The test is often repeated at intervals or after any major events, and provides an accurate measurement of changes in the heart over time. The test takes about half an hour, and requires that you lie still while the probe is placed over various parts of the chest. It involves virtually no discomfort, risk or inconvenience.

Electrocardiogram: This is a test to examine the electrical activity of the heart, and can pick up heart rhythm disturbances, signs of a heart attack or a prior heart attack, and can give important clues about the nature of heart disease, especially in the case of coronary artery disease or electrical disturbances. It is extremely simple, takes five to ten minutes, and simply involves placing electrodes (a kind of a sticky button) on the arms, legs and chest, and recording the electrical signals into a computer.

Electrophysiologic study: This test is somewhat less frequently performed in patients with a recent heart attack, but is used to assess the electrical functioning of the heart, and is particularly useful when patients have had a history of heart rhythm disturbances or fainting. During the test, the doctors try to deliberately bring on a rapid or irregular heart rhythm by means of an electrode wire placed inside the heart from veins in the leg or neck, using a temporary pacemaker connected to the wires inside the heart. The risk of complications from this test is low, but it can occasionally result in rapid palpitations or even loss of consciousness.

Exercise tests: An exercise test is usually used to diagnose the presence and severity of *myocardial ischemia*, i.e., lack of blood flow to the heart muscle. It can also provide important information about physical conditioning, and the response of the heart rate to exercise stress, and is important to establish safe levels of physical exercise for patients about to begin rehabilitation. It involves being connected to an ECG machine, and walking on a treadmill at an increasingly rapid rate and with an increasing incline (i.e., up an increasingly steeper hill), such that by the end of it some patients may be jogging uphill. The exercise can also be performed on a stationary bicycle. Although the test can be uncomfortable, since it does involve hard physical work, and will lead to breathlessness, and may lead to chest pain, it is quite safe since it is done under close supervision.

Holter monitoring: This test is primarily used to diagnose heart rhythm disturbances, particularly to discover the cause of palpitations or dizziness. The state of the blood supply to the heart can also be examined with this test. It involves measuring the electrocardiogram for twenty-four or more hours, by means of a device something like a cassette recorder attached to the body by wires and several electrodes, much like an ECG. Patients wear this device for one or several days, and the heart's electrical signals are continuously transmitted to a cassette tape, which is subsequently played back into a computer, and all of the beats are analyzed. The test involves a few minutes of hookup, and patients then go about their normal everyday activities until the device is returned. A diary is provided so that patients may write down any symptoms that they have, in order that the heartbeat at the moment symptoms occur can be analyzed.

MUGA scan: "MUGA" stands for a *multi-gated nuclear angiogram*, and is a way of studying the pumping action of the heart by injecting a small amount of radioactive material and taking a picture of the heart muscle as it contracts. A very accurate calculation of the strength of contraction or beating of various portions of the heart muscle can be made, using a computer that records many heartbeats and averages the result. This test allows a precise measurement of the severity of heart damage after a heart attack. It involves minimal discomfort and virtually no risk.

Nuclear imaging: These are tests that assess blood flow to the heart muscle by injecting a small amount of a radioactive substance (*thallium* or *Cardiolite®*) intravenously, and then taking a picture using a special camera (*gamma counter*) to accurately measure blood flow to the heart. This imaging is often combined with either exercise stress (on a treadmill or an exercise bicycle) or stress using an infusion of a medication that can "stress" the heart, bringing out subtle abnormalities of blood flow. These tests are positive if there are areas in the heart that receive no blood flow (because they are scarred from a previous heart attack), or receive normal blood flow at rest but insufficient blood flow during stress, thus indicating narrowing of the arteries to the heart. These important tests can estimate accurately the amount of heart muscle that is threatened with damage due to insufficient blood supply, and can help doctors decide if medication, angioplasty or bypass surgery is likely to be helpful. This test involves minimal discomfort because of the need for an intravenous, but is very safe.

SURGICAL PROCEDURES OFTEN PERFORMED ON PATIENTS WITH HEART DISEASE

Bypass surgery: Conceptually, bypass surgery is quite simple. It involves the fashioning of "detours" to route blood around sites of blockage in the arteries. Bypasses are made of veins taken from the leg or arteries from the chest wall; these are inserted or sewn into the heart arteries beyond the site of the most important blockages. Although bypass surgery is a fairly major operation, and usually involves placing the patient on a heart–lung machine while the heart is stopped so it can be operated on, the procedure is quite safe. These days, most patients remain in the hospital for five to seven days, unless complications occur, and need a relatively brief period of convalescence (four to six weeks) before resuming previous activities or even more strenuous activities than before, since their symptoms are usually much improved. In very recent developments, this surgery can sometimes be done without the patient being placed on a heart–lung machine, simplifying the procedure and making the recovery period shorter. After the surgery, there is discomfort at the incision sites, some inevitable fatigue, as well as the psychological adjustment of getting used to having had a fairly major heart operation. The risks of bypass surgery are generally quite low, with less than 5 percent having serious complications such as a heart attack or stroke, and no more than 2 or 3 percent with fatal complications.

While bypass surgery is very effective and usually leads to a marked improvement in symptoms, it is not curative, since the original hardening of the patient's arteries remains. Where veins are used to fashion the bypasses, the bypasses may begin to "give out" (become narrowed or blocked) after eight to twelve years or so, but where arteries are used they appear to last much longer.

The development and perfection of bypass surgery has truly revolutionized the treatment of heart disease. For those patients with severe narrowing of the arteries, especially if they have had prior heart attacks and have several vessels narrowed, the long-term outlook is very much better with bypass surgery than without. Importantly, most patients have an improvement in their ability to perform physical activities, and their general well-being improves after successful bypass surgery.

Coronary angioplasty: Sometimes also known as PTCA (*percutaneous transluminal coronary angioplasty*), this is a procedure to open narrowed arteries to the heart, by means of a deflated balloon that is threaded into the area of narrowing from a blood vessel in the groin; the balloon is inflated to a fairly high pressure to cause the area of narrowing to expand, thus restoring better blood flow. This procedure is successful in the vast majority of cases, although it does not cure the condition, since the deposits of calcium, scar tissue and cholesterol in the blood vessel wall remain but are displaced so that the opening in the artery is larger. Not all narrowings can be opened, or *dilated*, because of their dimensions and location, and not all of the attempts to perform this procedure are successful. However, many patients are eligible for this procedure, and when it is successful, it allows better blood flow and improves symptoms. Often chest pain disappears completely. There is a chance of recurring narrowings in the months following the procedure, however, and there are occasional complications. Fortunately, serious complications such as a heart attack or stroke are quite rare.

Coronary stenting: Since narrowing can recur in up to 30 percent of cases following initially successful angioplasty, cardiologists have developed *coronary stents*—small, delicate, cylindrical wire-mesh objects that can be inserted into an opened-up artery to hold it open, much like scaffolding. They are "folded up," then passed through the arteries to the site of previous blockage, where they "spring open" and hold the artery walls apart. With these ingenious devices, the chance of a blood vessel remaining open is much better and the long-term results are very good. These days, many patients who have angioplasty also receive one or several stents.

MEDICATIONS OFTEN PRESCRIBED FOR PATIENTS WITH HEART DISEASE

Angiotensin converting enzyme inhibitors (ACE inhibitors): These drugs lower blood pressure, and decrease the amount of work the heart needs to do to pump blood. The consequence of having a weak heart muscle (heart failure) is that sensors in the large blood vessels such as the aorta and the kidneys receive low blood flow. The body counteracts this consequence of poor cardiac performance by manufacturing a variety of hormones and other circulating substances that constrict blood vessels, raise blood pressure, and cause the kidneys to retain salt and water. This reaction is very similar to the sudden and massive "fight or flight response," which occurs during severe physical stress such as major injury or bleeding.

The defense mechanisms called into play when the heart is pumping weakly, normally intended to defend the body against sudden severe stresses, are inappropriate, and even harmful, when dealing with long-term continuous stresses, such as those caused by permanent weakness of the heart's pumping action.

These defense mechanisms result in overactivity of the hormone *angiotensin*, which causes blood vessels to constrict and raises blood pressure. With a healthy heart, this would not be much of a problem, but in a patient with a weak heart muscle, an increase in blood pressure causes the heart to work excessively hard and fail more rapidly. Other defense mechanisms include increased stickiness of blood platelets, and activation of the blood-clotting mechanism, all of which makes it more likely that clotting will occur inside blood vessels. The kidneys retain salt and water, and therefore there is an excess of salt and water in the body. This causes an increase in the amount of blood to be pumped by the heart, and also increases the heart's workload. A failing heart has difficulty pumping this extra amount of blood, and hence the need to restrict salt intake and use "water pills" (*diuretics*), to allow the kidneys to get rid of extra salt and water in heart failure.

ACE inhibitors are drugs that directly prevent an excess of the active form of angiotensin. This drug is very effective at lowering blood pressure, and is particularly effective in patients with heart failure. There is now excellent evidence from a large number of research studies that blood-pressure lowering with ACE inhibitors preserves the heart's pumping functions, reduces death rates and improves quality of life in patients with heart failure. The drug should probably be used by most patients with either substantial heart muscle weakness or a recent heart attack. Although it is not intuitive, even to some doctors, that "low blood pressure" is better than "normal blood pressure" in patients with heart failure, most patients with moderate or substantial heart damage in fact feel better and live longer if their blood pressure is lower than the average. Patients and families thus need to be aware that their blood pressure while taking these drugs may be as low as 100/70 (the higher number is the *systolic* and the lower number the *diastolic* pressure). The normal average blood pressure is about 120/80, although this tends to climb with age, so most sixty- or seventy-year-olds in Western society have blood pressure in the range of 140–150/80–90 mmHg (millimeters of mercury). The desirable blood pressure on ACE inhibitors is thus a fair bit lower than average. (Remember, there is no harm, but there is benefit, when patients with heart failure have blood pressure at this level.)

In patients who cannot take ACE inhibitors (as is very occasionally the case because of kidney malfunction or cough caused by these medications), other drugs that lower blood pressure, known as "afterload reducing agents" (drugs that lower blood pressure by dilating blood vessels), can be used. These drugs include *angiotensin 2 receptor antagonists*, varying forms of nitroglycerin (*nitrates*, see below) and *hydralazine*.

Importantly, habitual physical exercise also lowers blood pressure by helping blood vessels relax, and thus makes the job of the heart easier.

If a patient takes more ACE inhibitors or similar drugs than necessary, blood pressure may fall too low and cause dizziness or lightheadedness, especially on standing up quickly. This is not dangerous, but may indicate the need to cut back on the dose. Patients with heart diseases require very careful regulations of their medications. The medications discussed in this section are all helpful, and many are literally life-saving or life-prolonging. However, their use requires careful monitoring and a certain amount of expertise in the selection of the best drug and the best dose for a particular patient. For this reason, there are advantages to patients to seeing, at least on occasion, physicians expert in the care of heart disease, including particular complications of heart disease, such as cardiologists who have special expertise and experience in the treatment of heart failure (see page 182).

Aspirin and like drugs: These drugs prevent platelets from sticking together. The oldest and best studied is aspirin (*acetylsalicylic acid* or *ASA*), long known to be an effective pain reliever and fever remedy. Aspirin is very effective in preventing heart attack and coronary-related death, especially in patients with prior heart attack or unstable angina. It should probably be given to most or all patients with coronary artery diseases unless they are allergic (rare).

ASA-like drugs such as *ticlopidine* and *clopidogrel* also prevent platelets from sticking together. All these drugs have been widely studied and are quite effective, although aspirin is the most commonly used because of its long history, ease of use and inexpensiveness. ASA does, however, cause occasional stomach upset, and even ulcers or bleeding from the lining of the stomach. Other, newer drugs appear to be even more effective at preventing platelets from sticking together and are very useful in preventing heart attacks and prolonging life in patients with unstable angina or at high risk for clotting, but they may cause more bleeding.

Beta blockers: Beta blockers are a family of drugs that counteract the effects of adrenaline and other similar hormones on the body. They are extremely effective in reducing the workload of the heart, treating chest pain or discomfort, lowering high blood pressure and preventing the recurrence of heart attacks or death after an initial attack. These are undoubtedly the best "all-purpose drugs" for patients with coronary heart disease. Why are they so useful?

Simply put, the "sympathetic nervous system" of the human body uses adrenaline as one of its main "defense tools" in the "fight or flight response" to severe physical stresses. While this response was essential for our primitive forebears and their perilous hunter-gatherer culture, in modern Western society, we face very different kinds of stresses, for which we may be biologically poorly adapted. Modern life is marked by continuous low-grade stress, such as that produced by crowding in urban environments, dealing with complex social structures, multiple conflicting demands on our time and attention, and ambiguous social situations where there is no single right course of action. The adrenergic nervous system, which was adapted to deal with sudden bursts or pulses of adrenaline at infrequent intervals, is very poorly adapted to defending against the stresses of modern society. Chronic low-grade activation of the adrenergic nervous system is, in fact, harmful. It is for this reason that beta blockers, which directly counteract the effects of adrenaline on the heart, may be so useful. Beta blockers slow the heartbeat, slightly weaken the force of contraction of the heart, and lower blood pressure. Although it might seem that a drug that can even slightly weaken the pumping action of an already damaged heart would be harmful, in fact beta blockers seem to protect a weakened heart from further damage and weakening. Most patients with coronary heart disease should be on one of many different kinds of beta blockers available. Their main side effect is fatigue, and occasionally excessive slowing of the heartbeat.

A word about heart rate is important here. Although beta blockers can slow the heartbeat quite a bit in some cases, to as low as fifty beats per minute or below, this is not dangerous, and, in fact, if patients do not suffer from undue fatigue or lightheadedness, it is probably beneficial. It is useful to imagine that one has a certain number of heartbeats available over a lifetime, which can be used up "quickly" or slowly, depending on how fast the heart is beating.

In general, the slower the heartbeat, the better off you are—and this is certainly true after a heart attack, when patients with a fast heartbeat have a poorer outlook than those with a slow heartbeat. Although the heartbeat is increased *during* exercise, patients who exercise regularly, including those with heart disease, will have in general a slower heartbeat at rest, which of course accounts for most of the hours of the day.

Drugs that act on the clotting mechanism ("blood thinners"): As mentioned above, the "final straw" in a heart attack is the formation of a clot inside the blood vessel. The blood-clotting mechanism is activated by injury inside the blood vessel wall, much as blood will clot when you cut yourself because of injury to the skin and the blood vessels underneath it. Clotting is caused by the activation of blood elements called *platelets,* which stick together to plug holes in the blood vessel wall, and then by the formation of a blood clot itself, which is a complex lattice of proteins that otherwise circulate in the blood. In the case where the damage is inside the blood vessel itself, these clots can block up the inside of the blood vessel (known as the *lumen*), and are highly undesirable. One can counteract these processes by interfering with the action of the blood platelets, preventing them from sticking together; preventing blood from clotting by interfering with the proteins that lead to the clot itself; or dissolving the clots after they have been formed.

Heparin is an agent given intravenously that prevents clots themselves from forming, and has been long used and is very effective in "acute coronary syndromes," such as unstable angina or heart attack. The drug is used with most patients who arrive at the hospital with prolonged chest pain, and newer types of heparin may also be used on an outpatient basis, injected under the skin. Heparin is very effective in preventing heart attacks and some of their complications, but is used only for the short term and usually in the hospital. The dose needs to be carefully regulated by means of frequent blood tests, and it is common to have bruising when heparin is administered. Although this is unsightly, it is usually not dangerous or painful.

Warfarin (perhaps better known by its brand name, Coumadin®) is a blood thinner taken daily by mouth and is extremely useful in treating many cardiac disorders. It is especially helpful in preventing strokes in predisposed patients, most particularly those with *atrial fibrillation*. It is also used to prevent clotting in patients with artificial heart valves and for some patients with a prior heart attack, especially if there is marked enlargement of the heart or evidence for clot formation in the heart. Patients on warfarin require regular blood tests, usually weekly or every two weeks, to regulate the "thinness" of the blood. This test is extremely important since the effect of the drug can vary over time with changes in diet, activity, or even the seasons. For example, green leafy vegetables and other foods that contain vitamin K tend to counteract the effect of warfarin and, as the diet changes, so can the drug's effects. The blood tests very accurately indicate the effectiveness of the drug, and the result is expressed as the *international normalized ratio* (*INR*), which can be thought of as the time taken for the blood of patients on this drug to clot with respect to normal blood. The value in patients on no drugs is 1, and the desired value for most patients on warfarin is between 2 and 3. Values less than 2 therefore indicate blood that is clotting too rapidly ("insufficiently thin"), and values above 3 for most patients indicate excessive thinness of the blood (exceptions include patients with plastic and metal heart valves, and some others). Your doctor will tell you what INR value is ideal for you. It needs to be stressed that patients should not take warfarin without close medical supervision. Many medications can interfere with the action of warfarin, and thus your doctor and your pharmacist should be made aware of all medications you are taking.

Thrombolytics, or "clot busters," have been in use for about ten years to minimize the amount of heart damage after a heart attack. The original clot buster was called *streptokinase*, and most patients now get a more effective form called *tPA*. This drug acts to dissolve a clot that has already formed, allowing blood flow in a completely blocked artery to be at least partially restored. These drugs are very effective, especially when given early after the onset of a heart attack, restoring blood flow in over 75 percent of cases. However, to be most effective, they need to be administered as early as possible after the onset of a heart attack, preferably within the first few hours. Clot busters are generally quite safe, although they may cause bleeding in less than 1 percent of patients. The effectiveness of these drugs is the main reason why it is so important to go to the hospital if you have had chest pain, tightness or discomfort that has lasted more than thirty minutes, especially if it has not gotten better with nitroglycerin (by spray or tablets under the tongue).

Calcium antagonists: These are drugs that block the entry of calcium into heart cells, and open up the heart's and other blood vessels, slightly weakening the pumping action of the heart. They lower blood pressure and are quite effective at diminishing the frequency and severity of attacks of angina, especially if chest pain or discomfort occurs at rest or with minimal provocation. The drugs cause very few side effects except for rare headache or ankle swelling. However, there is not good evidence that calcium antagonists, unlike beta blockers, prolong life or prevent heart attacks. Nevertheless, they are frequently used in cases of severe or frequent chest pain or discomfort.

Cholesterol-lowering drugs: Many drugs can effectively lower cholesterol. As detailed below, cholesterol lowering is one of the cornerstones of the prevention of recurring heart attacks in many patients. The most effective of these drugs are known as *statins* (technically, *HMG CoA reductase inhibitors*), substances that decrease the manufacture of cholesterol by the body, in particular "bad cholesterol," carried in so-called low-density lipoproteins (LDL). These drugs can lower blood cholesterol very substantially, much more powerfully than even the most stringent diets. As well, they are extremely effective at lowering the incidence of death, recurring heart attack and other heart problems in many patients following a heart attack, especially patients with high cholesterol. Recent research studies have also shown that people with "normal cholesterol" who have had a heart attack can also benefit from these drugs. It appears that the ideal cholesterol level for patients with a history of coronary heart disease is in the low-normal, and even below-normal, range. The target value, for the technically minded, is a *low-density lipoprotein* cholesterol (which is only part of all the cholesterol in the blood) of less than 2.6 mmol/L (equivalent to 98.8 mg/dL). It should be noted that blood cholesterol is reported by most laboratories as "total cholesterol," for which the normal value is 200 mg/dL or 5.2 mmol/L.

Statins are quite safe, rarely causing muscle or liver problems, but patients can be monitored for both and such problems are reversible if the drug is stopped. The drug is prescribed for lifelong use.

Other cholesterol-lowering drugs such as *fibrates* and their derivatives are used in particular patient groups such as diabetics, and are probably also effective but less clearly well established to lower heart attack rates than are the *statins.*

Digoxin: Digoxin, a drug derived from a species of the foxglove plant, has been used to treat heart disease for many centuries. It slightly strengthens the beating of the heart, and slows heart rate, especially in the irregular heartbeat condition known as *atrial* *fibrillation* (see page 157). Although it does not prolong life, it can decrease breathlessness and improve well-being in patients with heart failure, and can modestly reduce palpitations in atrial fibrillation. It can have side effects at higher doses, however, and its dose needs to be monitored regularly.

Diuretics ("water pills"): Many patients with heart muscle weakness develop heart failure, as detailed above. Extra salt and water retained in the body can cause bloating, ankle swelling, and especially shortness of breath, because of an increased amount of salt and water in the blood vessels in the lungs. In such patients, excess salt in the diet—for example, from salty foods such as pickles, peanuts, pretzels, potato chips, and so on—can cause a significant worsening of symptoms. Although it is important to be careful not to add too much salt at the table, most salt in the diet comes from the "hidden" sources, in packaged, canned and prepared foods. As a general rule, low-salt diets focus on fresh foods such as fruits, vegetables, pasta and meats.

In addition to limiting salt intake, many patients with heart failure need diuretics, which are medications that cause the kidney to allow more salt and water to pass into the urine and be eliminated from the body. These medications may be inconvenient to take since they cause frequent urination, but have very important benefits in increasing well-being and decreasing breathlessness. Patients with heart failure are often instructed to weigh themselves fairly frequently; if there is a sudden weight gain, such as a pound per day or more over a few days, usually this indicates extra salt and water being retained by the body and may indicate the need for additional diuretics.

Nitroglycerin: Nitroglycerin has been around for a long time, and is a compound that opens up or dilates blood vessels, including blood vessels to the heart. Nitroglycerin and its family of drugs called *nitrates* are available as under-the-tongue tablets or as a spray to be used on the back of the throat. These drugs are very effective for the short-term relief of chest discomfort, although the effects are very brief. Nitrates are also available as longer-lasting tablets that are taken by mouth, or applied to the skin in the form of patches. The main side effect is headache.

Since nitrates are very effective in the short-term relief of chest discomfort caused by insufficient blood supply to the heart (*myocardial ischemia*), patients should not feel restraint in using them as often as necessary. If, however, chest discomfort persists after three nitro tablets or sprays five to ten minutes apart, patients should proceed to the nearest emergency department or consult with their doctors. Nitro spray can also be used *prior* to intended exercise; for example, before walks or other activities expected to cause angina.

General advice about medications

Many heart patients take five, six, or even more medications every day for a variety of reasons. The most common of these medications are listed above. Although it may seem "unnatural" and frustrating to have to take this many medications, each of them has proven benefits in prolonging life or improving well-being. Patients who require multiple medications are not necessarily "sicker" than those who require fewer medications, and you should look at medications as your friends rather than your enemies.

Despite their being a nuisance to take, inconvenient and expensive, there is absolutely no advantage to not taking medications recommended by your doctors. Many patients adopt the attitude that they are not really "pill takers" and try to "tough it out" with respect to their symptoms. In the case of heart disease (unlike in many other chronic conditions, such as arthritis), most of the medications doctors prescribe are truly life-prolonging, and protect you in a way that diet, exercise and other nondrug treatments cannot. This does not mean that drug therapy cannot be supplemented by changes in diet and exercise; rather, it means that the two need to be allowed to work together. For example, a low-salt, low-fat diet, as well as exercise, can lower blood pressure. It is rare, however, that these measures alone can restore normal levels in a patient with high blood pressure, although they work extremely well in concert with a regimen of medications. The same can be said of cholesterol-lowering therapy; even very strict low-fat, low-cholesterol diets decrease cholesterol only modestly, and in very many patients these need to be supplemented by drugs that lower cholesterol.

Getting the most from your medications requires that you take them exactly as prescribed. Surprisingly, as many as half of patients do not follow this advice, for many reasons, including forgetfulness, the cost of their medications, and, perhaps most important, the failure of doctors and caregivers to emphasize that medications must be taken exactly as directed. There is some evidence that patients who understand why they are taking their medications and understand the nature of their illness and the benefit of medications, can be faithful to their medication regimen.

There are a number of things you can do to make sure you follow instructions for taking your medication. First, be sure that you understand precisely why you are taking each medication and try, if possible, to remember its name. Second, make taking your medications habitual; for example, take them just before breakfast, just before bedtime, or at other times of day when you have a predictable schedule. If your medicine bottle is close to your toothbrush, you will be more likely to remember to take your pills every time you brush your teeth. There are some very helpful aids available in pharmacies to help you remember to take your medications, including special pillboxes where all the medications you need for a particular day or even a week are placed in small compartments. If you miss a dose, you will then be able to see immediately which dose you missed, and what you need to take at the next dose interval. Electronic gadgets, such as automatic timers and alarms, can be useful for the more mechanically inclined. If you miss a dose of medication, it is generally not a serious thing; for most pills you should simply take the next dose as scheduled, but do not pile the skipped dose on top of your next scheduled dose.

You should carry with you, at all times, a list of the pills you are taking, including the chemical names, and the dosages. This is extraordinarily important to have whenever you visit your doctor, so that your dose regimen can be properly recorded, but is also important to have with you in case of emergency.

YOUR TEAM OF PROFESSIONALS

ON YOUR JOURNEY of recovery, you will encounter many caregivers. It is useful to have an understanding of the kind of training and expertise they have so that you can benefit fully from those who will help you. *Doctors* are individuals who have graduated from a medical school with a degree as *Doctor of Medicine*, and then have gone on to do *postgraduate training*. These days, most doctors pursue specialized training in a particular field. This field may be *family medicine*, in which case doctors get two or three years of special training in looking after patients in the community. Young doctors nowadays get more extensive and longer training, and develop substantial expertise in the treatment of such common conditions as heart attack, high blood pressure, diabetes and stroke. A family doctor with whom you have a connection is especially important in helping you and your family deal with the non-hospital-based part of your care, which includes lifestyle changes, monitoring of medications, and the psychological and vocational consequences of illness.

Other doctors become specialists in *internal medicine*, which generally requires four or five years of training in hospitals. Much of this training will be in diseases of the *cardiovascular system*, chiefly the heart. *Cardiology* is a *subspecialty* of internal medicine, and *cardiologists* will have a total of six or more years of specialized training after medical school, three or more of them specifically in diseases of the heart. At the end of this training period, cardiologists can be considered experts in the treatment of all aspects of heart disease.

However, recent developments in techniques, procedures and treatments for heart disease have led to the growth of *subsubspecialties* of internal medicine, or subspecialties of cardiology. Physicians developing such specific expertise have an additional two, or even more, years of training in a subspecialty, and thus are highly qualified in their particular area of interest. For example, there are cardiologists particularly interested in heart failure and its treatment; those who develop particular technical proficiency in procedures such as coronary angiography and angioplasty; those with special expertise in the performance and interpretation of tests such as nuclear cardiology, or echocardiography (ultrasound); and those with special expertise in electrophysiology (the study of heart rhythm disturbances). In virtually all university-based teaching hospitals, and some community hospitals, there will be cardiologists with such sub-subspecialized training and expertise. Although not all patients with heart disease have the need for or access to such highly specialized care, these cardiologists are an important resource to family doctors, internists and other cardiologists, both with respect to advice about individual patients and in keeping the medical community abreast of the latest changes in treatment for cardiac patients. For many patients with moderately serious or serious heart disease, it is very useful to have at least a consultation with a cardiologist or a subspecialist in one of the cardiac disciplines in order to help the primary treating physicians make a plan for ongoing investigation and care. If patients are not responding well to treatment, or have particular difficulties, the treating physicians should not feel insulted or slighted if a consultation with a sub-subspecialist is requested.

Sub-subspecialists are very often engaged in research in their particular discipline, which allows them access to new or innovative treatments somewhat earlier than the general medical profession. These physicians will often be actively engaged in doing research studies, and they may approach you for participation in one of these studies (see below).

Dietitians have had extensive training in nutrition, diet and the effects of food on illness and health. They have particular expertise unique to their discipline, and they are an extremely important part of the multidisciplinary team looking after heart patients.

Exercise physiologists have particular training from a university in the types, results of and techniques of exercise, and usually help plan and supervise exercise programs for patients with a variety of illnesses, including cardiac disease. They are often instrumental in constructing exercise programs for cardiac rehabilitation centers.

Psychologists often work closely together with cardiac teams or cardiac rehabilitation centers to help in patient education and to help patients with the motivation and techniques necessary for change in lifestyle and behavior, and can deal with particular psychological problems that often arise in heart patients, such as anxiety, depression and feelings of helplessness. They often coordinate particular treatment programs such as group therapy, stress or relaxation therapy, and many offer individual psychotherapy. *Psychiatrists* are medical doctors with extensive training in psychology, behavior and mental illness, and often work as consultants to cardiologists or cardiology rehabilitation programs.

Nurses are perhaps the most important professionals looking after patients with heart disease. They are often the "glue" that holds the multidisciplinary team together. The first and last contact in the hospital, often in outpatient clinics, and in rehabilitation programs will be a registered nurse. Nowadays, nurses receive university training in nursing followed by clinical training in a hospital setting. They are experts in not only hands-on caring for patients, but also in helping patients deal with the burden of their illness, including its physical, social, psychological, emotional and financial dimensions. In most cases, nurses will get to know their patients personally and are more accessible on that level than are doctors, and are an extremely important resource for you and your family for advice, encouragement and for help in taking in the large amount of information that you will be exposed to, especially during an in-hospital stay.

MEDICAL RESEARCH

JUST ABOUT EVERYTHING we know in modern medical science is the result of research, usually performed over many years by many individuals in different countries. Modern medicine is vastly different from traditional sciences, such as physics and chemistry, and from other disciplines, such as philosophy. Whereas in these areas individual thinkers or scientists make important observations which may be subsequently observed to be true or not true over time, in modern medical science, developments occur "bit by bit" in an unpredictable pattern, and are very rarely the result of one great mental leap made by one individual. For example, the development of "clot busters," an extraordinarily important event in the treatment of patients with acute heart attack, and one that is undoubtedly associated with dramatic patient benefit, was the result of decades of research by many different individuals in many different disciplines (including studies of blood clotting; biochemical studies of the drugs; understanding of the relationship between the clotting system, blood vessel wall, and various physical stresses). Clot busters, like all other current treatments, were finally proven to be effective in *controlled clinical trials*, which are extensive tests of a particular medication or treatment done in patients with the disease in question.

Patients with heart disease and the general lay public are these days bombarded with information about treatments or substances which are alleged to be beneficial in treating heart disease. These include vitamins, diet, drugs, treatments such as chelation therapy, as well as more traditional treatments such as bypass surgery and angioplasty. Although any of these treatments can in theory be effective, and it is natural that patients will be drawn to the simplest, cheapest and least complicated of these therapies, we can unfortunately not be assured that any of these treatments is truly effective until it is properly tested. For medical researchers, such proper testing requires that the treatment in question be compared to some other treatment, usually a *placebo* (an inactive substance), thus allowing an unambiguous comparison of the *test treatment* to *no treatment* in order to eliminate any biases, which are inevitable when human beings, with all of their expectations and frailties, judge human health or disease. Almost all trials need to be *double-blind*; in other words, neither the caregivers nor the patient is aware of the nature of the treatment he or she is receiving. In practice, this means that a very large group of patients with the disease in question—in our particular example, an acute heart attack—had to be given either the active clot-busting agent or a placebo, and the patients and their doctors and nurses did not know which was actually being administered to any given individual. Patients were all monitored very closely, and at the end of some time period, such as one or two months, the results were compared. In this way, it was proven beyond doubt that patients who had received clot busters lived longer and had less heart damage than those who had not received them. It is important to emphasize that, in the absence of such rigorously performed and very expensive and time-consuming research studies, we can never be really sure whether or not a treatment is truly effective. This is true in almost all situations, unless an illness is usually fatal in the absence of treatment (e.g., appendicitis or severe pneumonia). Since most patients with heart disease recover to some extent even without treatment, such blinded studies are absolutely essential if true benefit from a particular treatment is to be proven.

Therapies which are now universally accepted as being beneficial, such as ASA, beta blockers after heart attack, and treatments to lower blood pressure in patients with high blood pressure, have all been verified to be effective in such clinical trials. Refinement in drug therapy of course continues and has even accelerated in recent years. There are thus many new clot-busting agents available for testing, or new treatments for high blood pressure, which potentially promise to be more effective, safer, or simpler to take and use. Each of these needs to be compared to some standard treatment, usually the currently available therapy in general clinical use. Patients with almost any form of heart disease may be approached to participate in such clinical trials. The usual process is that a patient is identified as having the particular illness or characteristics ideally suited for the testing of a new treatment or procedure. Patients will then be approached to participate in such research trials, and it will be stressed that their participation is entirely voluntary.

Although many patients or their families have justifiable reservations about being an experimental subject, or a "guinea pig," participating in these studies may give you a chance to receive a new, potentially more effective or safer treatment. You will also have the less obvious but important benefit of being monitored and cared for by a team of very expert individuals. Perhaps not surprisingly, patients in such clinical trials, even if they receive the inactive substance, or placebo, generally have better outcomes than apparently comparable patients who are not part of clinical trials. There is of course no guarantee that the experimental treatment will be effective, nor even that it will be safe. All treatments unfortunately carry some risk of causing harm, whether they are experimental or not; simply, the risk from experimental therapies is less well known although it may not necessarily be higher. For example, plain old ASA can often cause irritation of the stomach lining, and even bleeding ulcers in the stomach, potentially with serious consequences. The fact that these traditional side effects are known and understood does not make them less serious.

The other reason that patients may wish to participate in clinical trials is the knowledge that such tests are the only way to establish the effectiveness of new treatments or procedures, which can potentially be of great benefit to future patients with the illness. In this way, patients who participate in such trials are helping fellow patients have full access to potentially life-saving treatments in future years.

In practice, patients approached for participation in clinical trials will be given information about the study (the *trial*), including a *consent form*, which details all of the study procedures, potential risks and potential benefits. Participation in any such research study is voluntary, and patients should never be coerced overtly, or subtly, to consent. Patients also need to know that they can withdraw from studies at any time if they change their mind about participation. Many patients, however, find that the reasons to participate outweigh the reasons not to, and the medical profession has been fortunate in having outstanding cooperation from patients in performing this kind of research. As a result, there have been a number of gigantic studies in the past decade involving many tens of thousands of patients, which has allowed cardiologists and other doctors to be much more confident than they otherwise could have been in their assessment of the efficacy of certain treatments.

RISK FACTORS FOR CORONARY HEART DISEASE

Coronary heart disease can develop in anyone, without there necessarily being some known cause. However, there are many factors that are known to make it more likely that hardening of the arteries (*atherosclerosis*) will develop in a given individual. In no particular order, these include high cholesterol levels in the blood, current or recent smoking, diabetes, high blood pressure, a family history of coronary heart disease, obesity, a sedentary lifestyle, and possibly a psychological profile (formerly characterized as "type A," but more likely to be angry, hostile or depressed).

It is important to understand that these *risk factors* (discussed alphabetically below) are not necessarily present in every patient with coronary heart disease. In this sense, it is not valid to see patients as causing their "heart disease" or being directly responsible for it. Many patients with coronary heart disease do not have a known risk factor, and the disease thus seems to arise "out of the blue." However, many of these factors are at least partially modifiable, and bear discussion.

Cholesterol: There are many excellent resources for patients and families to find out about cholesterol, and its importance in heart disease. We provide only a very brief summary here. Cholesterol is a natural substance found in the blood and body tissues, which is necessary for the body's normal functioning. Most of the cholesterol in the blood is manufactured by the liver, and does not come directly from the diet. However, a diet high in fats, particularly so-called *saturated fats* (found in animal products, whole milk or butter, and certain plant oils) leads to a higher cholesterol level in the blood since more is manufactured by the liver. Since cholesterol is a form of fat, and since it doesn't mix with the water in the blood, much as oil and vinegar do not readily mix in a salad dressing, cholesterol is transported or ferried around in the blood in transport modules called *lipoproteins.* Cholesterol packaged in *low-density lipoproteins* is so-called bad cholesterol, since it is this type of transport module that carries the cholesterol to blood vessel walls, where it may settle, ultimately causing and contributing to hardening of the arteries. To simplify, cholesterol packaged in *high-density lipoproteins* is more likely to be carried away from blood vessel walls, and thus this carrier transport can ferry cholesterol away from blood vessels where it does the most damage. *High-density lipoproteins* are thus "good cholesterol."

There is now very clear scientific evidence that the higher the blood cholesterol, the greater the risk of developing coronary heart disease. The level of blood cholesterol in a given person is largely genetically determined, but can be slightly to moderately altered by diet. However, even with the most stringent diet, blood cholesterol can usually not be lowered by much more than about 20 percent.

Recent scientific studies have shown that patients with high cholesterol, or even so-called normal cholesterol (that is, at the average for Western society), can reduce their risk of heart attack or death by taking cholesterol-lowering drugs known as *statins.* Although it seems less artificial to modify the diet in order to lower cholesterol, there should be no shame or guilt attached to taking a drug to lower cholesterol, especially when such drugs are undoubtedly effective and rarely cause side effects. It should be remembered that taking cholesterol-lowering drugs is not a license to eat high-fat foods; rather, such drugs should be part of a treatment program that includes a sensible low-fat diet and exercise.

How does cholesterol wreak havoc in the arteries?

Although we are not entirely certain how it happens, cholesterol is probably deposited inside the cells lining the artery walls, called *endothelial cells*, where they can go through a chemical process known as *oxidation* and become irritants that stimulate the blood vessel walls to essentially form a scar. This scarring includes deposits of extra muscle cells, scar cells (fibrous tissue) and calcium. Although "hardening of the arteries" eventually leads to precisely what the term implies—rock-hard and stonelike blockages of the arteries—initially this process involves soft, fatty deposits inside blood vessel walls that are prone to tear or rupture, leading to clot formation and a rapid increase in the severity of blockage. This is probably why cholesterol lowering, especially the marked cholesterol lowering that can be achieved with drugs, can lead to very rapid diminishing of the risk of heart attack or death, although the deposits themselves may have been building up for years or decades. The important conclusion from recent research studies is that it is never too late to lower your cholesterol, and that the benefits can be seen quite quickly once treatment is started. All patients with a history of coronary heart disease should have their cholesterol measured, and treated to lower the cholesterol level in the blood if it is too high. The more risk factors a patient has, the more important it becomes to achieve and maintain an ideal cholesterol level.

Diabetes: Diabetes is a very common disorder that results from inability of the body to use sugar in the blood (the main form of sugar is called *glucose*), one of the main sources of energy for the body to perform its functions. Glucose from the blood enters muscles and other tissues under the influence of the hormone *insulin*, which comes from the pancreas gland. Diabetes is a condition in which the glucose in the blood cannot be taken up by muscles and other tissues, either because there is an insufficient amount of insulin released by the pancreas, or because the insulin that is available cannot work effectively.

Diabetes is commonly thought of as an illness in children or young individuals, who usually need insulin by injection one or several times daily, because their pancreas produces no insulin at all. This severe form of diabetes is fortunately relatively uncommon. Very much more common is another type, known as *type II diabetes*; patients with this type do not usually require insulin by injection, although they need to take drugs by mouth to lower their blood-sugar levels. This more common form of diabetes is a very major risk factor for coronary heart disease, and is closely related to obesity, or being overweight. A set of conditions, including excess weight, high blood pressure, diabetes, and high blood fats known as *triglycerides*, has been termed *syndrome X*. Patients with this syndrome are extremely prone to coronary heart disease, and the condition improves markedly with exercise, weight loss and a low-fat diet. Contrary to popular belief, for most diabetics the most important dietary advice is not to restrict sugar, but to maintain a normal weight and to limit fat intake. Many diabetics have only slightly elevated blood sugars, and may be unaware that they are diabetic unless they are specifically tested.

Diet: The question of diet has received much discussion in both the scientific and the lay press. There are many books entirely devoted to diets or dietary advice for patients with heart disease, and it is not our intention to give an exhaustive review of the relationship between diet and heart disease.

In our view, attention to diet is an important component of the journey of recovery from heart disease. However, diet alone cannot cure and, for almost all patients, cannot reverse heart disease; we do not feel it is realistic to expect that any diet, however stringent, can by itself cure or reverse hardening of the arteries. This is especially true in the "real-life practices" that we see among our patients, most of whom do not have the time, resources and opportunity to follow the very particular and sometimes stringent diets occasionally advocated. Most North Americans find a very low fat diet unpalatable, and it is unrealistic to expect most patients to adhere strictly to a diet very different from the one they have been accustomed to for perhaps fifty or more years. Although a great deal of emphasis has been placed on reducing the amount of cholesterol in the diet, by avoiding red meats, eggs, whole milk and other cholesterol-rich foods, most of the cholesterol in the blood is manufactured by the liver and does not come from dietary sources. In addition, the best way to lower cholesterol in the blood is to limit the *fat* content of the diet, rather than limiting cholesterol alone.

An important aspect of paying attention to one's diet is the opportunity for weight loss, which not only leads to a reduction in the risk of development or worsening of heart disease, but improves well-being, self-image and exercise tolerance. We feel that the best way to change one's diet is to develop a different relationship with food, rather than to be excessively vigilant about the calorie and fat and cholesterol content of every bite or every meal. In general, the healthiest diets are the ones that are rich in fresh fruits and vegetables, bread or other grains, and skim or low-fat milk or milk products. These diets will include less meat than most North Americans regularly consume, and definitely less fat. In general, prepared foods (especially those served in fast-food restaurants), desserts and snack foods are high in fat and calories. The best example of a healthy diet is that taken by people in the Mediterranean region, and scientific studies have shown that this diet reduces coronary events. The Mediterranean diet primarily uses olive oil as its source of fat, and contains a lot of pasta, grains, fruits and vegetables, and fish, and relatively little meat and convenience foods.

From a practical perspective, limiting between-meal snacks, and cutting intake of meats and rich sauces (containing butter or oil), is a good start to a heart-healthy diet. It is important that diet be understood as a lifelong habit of healthy eating, and not as a temporary change in eating habits designed to lead to weight loss alone. Heart disease takes many decades to develop, as we stated before, and dietary changes cannot be expected to alter this process very quickly. In fact, it may take many years, or even longer, for the benefits of a change in diet to be observed.

Specific aspects of diet or dietary supplements deserve mention. Patients who eat fish more often appear to have a lower incidence of heart disease, especially those who eat fatty fish such as salmon. It is not clear if it is the fish itself that is protective, or whether these patients in general tend to have better diets. Fish-oil supplements, available in capsule form from health food stores, have been advocated by some to protect against heart disease, but in our opinion the evidence is inconclusive. We do not recommend fish-oil supplementation to our patients, although the risks are probably small. Vitamin E, present in vegetables (especially green vegetables) and other foods, is an antioxidant and may protect against heart disease. Again, the evidence for this is inconclusive, and large scientific studies are being conducted at this moment to see if vitamin E supplements can prevent the worsening of heart disease. Until the results of these studies are available, we do not generally recommend vitamin E, although the risks of taking it are probably quite small.

A great deal of research has been done on the effects of *alcohol consumption* on heart disease. Although no research study has ever truly compared alcohol as a "drug" and a "placebo" in the manner discussed above, it seems quite clear that individuals who drink moderate amounts of alcohol (generally defined as two or at most three standard drinks (a bottle of beer or a glass of wine) per day have a lower likelihood of developing heart disease than those who drink no alcohol or who drink higher amounts. Although there are theoretical reasons to believe that wine, especially red wine, may be more likely to be beneficial than other forms of alcohol, this is by no means clear from the research studies performed. Alcohol in any form is known to raise the level of "good cholesterol" (see page 189), and this may be the mechanism of its benefit. We do not advocate taking alcohol as a medicine or a drug, but would certainly agree that moderate alcohol consumption is not dangerous, if this is a habit you already have. It is very clear that alcohol consumption, especially in excess, carries potential health risks, most especially the risk of impairment in operating motor vehicles, the possibility of liver disease, and the enormous social and economic costs of alcoholism. The advice about alcohol is therefore not to be taken lightly. Nevertheless, if you find a glass or two of wine or a beer with your meals or on social occasions to be pleasant, we advise that you continue this practice.

The question of the effect of *caffeine* on coronary heart disease is not entirely settled. Although there is much folklore surrounding the effects of caffeine, which can definitely cause jitteriness, palpitations and anxiety if taken in large quantities, there is no clear reason to believe that caffeine is dangerous for the heart. It is extremely difficult to disentangle the effects of coffee from other factors that may influence heart disease, since individuals who drink a lot of coffee may be more likely to be anxious, for example, more likely to smoke, and may be likely to have a different diet than non–coffee drinkers. It is prudent to avoid very large amounts of caffeine, but the occasional cup of coffee is very unlikely to be harmful.

Exercise: Physical activity, or exercise, is possibly the most important component of both recuperation and rehabilitation in patients with coronary heart disease. We will not give extensive prescriptions for specific exercises, but it is important to have some knowledge of the types of exercise and the benefits of exercise.

First, exercise (to the cardiologist, at least) generally means *physical* activity, and is not the same as being "busy" or "rushing around." For example, a busy day at work, or a busy day at home, which may include making beds, housecleaning, cooking and shopping, may involve physical activity but usually does not qualify as exercise (although this type of activity may be beneficial to your heart, and certainly is better than inactivity). By exercise, we usually mean at least a single session of continuous activity lasting thirty to forty-five minutes, done at least three, and preferably four or five, times per week. This activity does not have to be a competitive sport, and does not have to be done at extremely high intensity for it to benefit your general well-being and your heart. For example, brisk walking, bicycling (on the road or on a stationary bicycle), swimming, slow jogging, as well as sports can provide the kind of benefits you need to make your heart work more efficiently. Usually, the activity is done at a sufficiently brisk pace to increase your heartbeat to more than 100 beats per minute, or to make you feel that you are working at least "somewhat" or "moderately" hard (though not necessarily "hard," "very hard," or "as hard as you can"). At the end of the period of exercise, you will generally be slightly tired, but should not be gasping for air, exhausted or so weak that you cannot immediately afterwards carry out ordinary, everyday activities. Although it is possible that health benefits may be obtained from briefer periods of exercise, most people find it inconvenient to exercise for only a few short minutes. Of course, it is very useful to be active when you can—for example, climbing one or two flights of stairs instead of taking the elevator, or walking to the store instead of taking the car—but by "exercise" we mean planned activity where expending energy is the object rather than only a means to an end.

Most people find that in order to achieve sustained benefit from an exercise program, a commitment to blocking out the time required for the activity is important. You may also find that others will exercise with you, such as new acquaintances in a rehabilitation program, family members, friends or individuals that you meet at, say, a cycling club, cross-country-skiing club, or walking or jogging club. The social aspects of exercise are extremely important, since friends and acquaintances will help motivate you to "stay on track" and not miss exercise sessions, and also provide you with a fellowship of shared goals as well as an accepting supportive network, both of which are very important to achieving heart health.

Why is exercise so important?

From prehistoric times up until very recently, humans had to be very physically active in order to survive. Before the invention of the internal-combustion engine, all of those chores that we now consider to be easy, such as finding and preparing food, building and caring for shelter, and visiting friends and neighbors, required a great deal of physical effort. These days, it is possible to lead a completely sedentary life, never having to walk further than a few hundred feet or to perform any physical activities whatsoever. Our bodies were not adapted to being inactive and, much like an automobile whose engine runs more smoothly when it is driven on the highway regularly, function better when they have been exercised regularly. The benefits of regular exercise are many. With regular exertion, the exercising muscles become more efficient at using the available blood supply from the heart, and the ability to exercise at higher intensity for longer periods of time improves. In other words, the more you do, the more you *can* do. Blood supply to exercising muscles will improve, and since the heart's job becomes easier, it is more efficient, and therefore can do more work, when you are fit. It is very important to remember that fitness does not require athletic ability, or championship-type intensity of effort. Simply walking briskly forty-five minutes a day, three to five times per week, will improve your fitness level, sometimes dramatically if you were very unfit before. The key is that the activity needs to be continuous. Exercise not only will get you into "better shape" and improve your well-being, but has numerous biological effects that together stall, and possibly even reverse, hardening of the arteries, as well as delay the general effects of aging on your heart and on your body.

The benefits include a lowering of blood cholesterol and reduction of blood fats, lowering of blood pressure, improving the ability of your body to use sugar if you are diabetic, making your blood less "sticky" and less liable to form clots, helping you burn calories (a vital part of any weight-loss program), helping you stop smoking if you are wishing to quit, and improving your general well-being and your outlook on life, which itself can make it easier for you to maintain a heart-healthy lifestyle.

There is very clear scientific evidence that a program of regular exercise, at least if done in the supervised setting of a rehabilitation clinic or other programs that may be done at home, will prolong life in patients following a heart attack. This benefit is manifested as a lower incidence of new heart attacks, death from heart weakness (*heart failure*), and even from serious rhythm disturbances of the heart.

So-called *resistance training*, or *isometric exercise*, which generally involves lifting weights or pushing against a resistance, as in calisthenics, is also beneficial. Such exercise improves strength, flexibility, well-being, and is an important part of any complete exercise program. It is a little less simple to undertake than the usual *isotonic exercises*, such as walking, bicycling and swimming, but all of these activities can be done with very little equipment and without the need for special facilities.

Before embarking on an exercise program, it is important that you check with your doctor or cardiologist to determine what level of exercise is safe for you (some amount of exercise will be safe for just about anybody), and to get some advice about the type, frequency and intensity of exercise that most suits your needs. Such advice is probably best obtained from an exercise rehabilitation clinic or a facility that specializes in exercise programs for heart patients, but once you complete the program you need not necessarily attend a clinic on a regular basis. Indeed, many successful programs use an exercise prescription for unsupervised exercise at home, combined with regular telephone follow-ups from the exercise center to make sure that you are performing the activity and not having particular problems.

As is true of other lifestyle changes, the key to starting and sticking to a program of regular exercise is commitment. If you treat exercise as an unpleasant chore, or something like a medication that you have to take because it will make you feel better although you really don't want to, you are not likely to be successful in the long term. Unfortunately, there is not much of a cultural reward in our society for regular noncompetitive physical activity, especially among young people. Although our society glorifies competitive sports and elite athletics, the kind of activity we are speaking about is done regularly, lifelong, and is generally noncompetitive (or "friendly" competitive). In order to be successful at lifelong exercise activity, you need to find an activity that you enjoy or one that you can learn to enjoy doing. Making this activity part of your routine, and finding other like-minded people to exercise with, are extremely important components of making exercise a part of your life rather than just a chore added to the many you already have to perform.

It is helpful to set realistic and modest goals for yourself, at least in the beginning. If you think you can walk a mile in, say, twenty minutes, then make it your goal to do this regularly, and then gradually increase slightly the pace or the distance, so that you may, for example, be walking a mile and a half in thirty minutes or two miles in forty minutes within a few weeks or months. If you are unable to exercise for days, or even weeks, you need not worry. Once the idea of exercising regularly is part of your regular habit, you will have no trouble returning to the activity.

You will also need to be patient. Your fitness level will not increase immediately, or dramatically, when you begin an exercise program. Rather, it will increase gradually, and even imperceptibly, at first, until you find that you can do much more than you did a few months ago, and in general have more energy. It may seem paradoxical that the more active you are, the more energy you have, but energy level is at least as much psychological as it is physical, and the more exercise you get, the better your sleep quality, the less anxious you will feel under stress, and the more you will be able to focus your energy on the goals you wish to achieve.

Family history: A propensity to develop coronary heart disease can be inherited. This is related, in part, to an inherited tendency to have high cholesterol levels, or abnormalities of the cholesterol "transportation system" that carries the particles around in your blood. Having this predisposition increases your risk of developing heart disease, especially at a younger age. The genetics of coronary heart disease are complicated. However, if there is a history of a first-degree relative having a heart attack or bypass surgery or angina before the age of sixty-five, and especially before the age of fifty (first-degree relatives include parents, siblings, grandparents, uncles, aunts and first cousins), you are probably at comparatively high risk.

This does not mean that you are predestined to suffer from coronary disease no matter what. This extra risk does mean that you need to take special care to avoid any other risk factors. For example, smoking is a problem for all individuals, but a disaster for those with a strong family history of coronary heart disease.

High blood pressure (*hypertension*): High blood pressure is a condition, often inherited, in which the pressure inside the walls of large arteries of the body is high. This is caused by excessive squeezing or *constriction* of the artery walls, faster blood flow than normal, or both. In many patients, this is made worse by salt excess, and it can certainly be made worse by being overweight. *Diabetes* is a very important risk factor for high blood pressure. Contrary to popular notions, physical or psychological stress, while they are undesirable, do not necessarily cause high blood pressure. Exercise or psychological stress can clearly elevate blood pressure for very short periods (during the initial stressful period), but are not known to cause high blood pressure in the long run. This means that, although stress reduction is very useful to improve quality of life, it will not by itself bring about a sufficient lowering of blood pressure to treat the condition. Similarly, weight loss and salt avoidance can lower blood pressure slightly, but for most patients drug therapy is required.

Untreated high blood pressure is a killer. It increases the narrowing of the arteries by injuring the wall of the blood vessels, and contributes to the development of *atherosclerosis*, or arterial hardening, and thus heart attacks. After long periods, high blood pressure causes strokes and kidney failure. There are many drugs available for high blood pressure, and their benefits in reducing these serious consequences are dramatic. Unfortunately, only about half of patients who have high blood pressure are treated in a consistent manner, and only half of those (one-quarter of the total of those with high blood pressure) receive adequate control. Adequate control has been defined as a blood pressure of less than 140/90 (the upper number is the systolic and the lower number is the diastolic), although recent research shows that the target blood pressure after treatment should be as low as 130/85, close to the normal average pressure of about 120/80.

High blood pressure cannot be cured. If you stop taking your blood-pressure medications, the pressure may remain normal for days, weeks, or even longer. Eventually it will creep back upwards, however; and as a result the treatment for high blood pressure is almost always lifelong. Since in rare cases, the causes of high blood pressure can be fully reversed, or are the result of other illnesses, consult with your doctor to be sure that you are thoroughly tested for these kinds of *secondary hypertension*.

Obesity: Being overweight is a large (pun intended) problem in North American society. It is probably equally related to the relatively high-fat diets that we consume, and our lack of physical activity. Although being overweight is not in itself the most important risk factor for coronary disease, it is associated with a higher likelihood of diabetes, high blood pressure, less physical activity, and thus at least indirectly with a higher likelihood of coronary heart disease. In addition, being overweight impairs quality of life, since it makes it more difficult to perform pleasurable physical activities such as walking or traveling, and since patients' self-image is improved by maintaining a normal weight. Achieving and maintaining a normal weight is a daunting and difficult task. We suggest to our patients that weight loss not be seen as an isolated goal in the process of cardiac recovery, but as part and parcel of increases in activity level, gradual but permanent changes in diet and modification of other risk factors. Slow, gradual weight loss is preferable to a sudden dramatic loss of weight, and this type of weight loss is more likely to be maintained in the long run.

Smoking: So much has been written about smoking that virtually all readers will be aware of its dangers, particularly to the heart. Fortunately, fewer and fewer individuals are now smoking, although regrettably there are too many young people, especially females, taking up the habit in this decade. Cigarette smoke increases the heart rate, constricts blood vessels, causes cholesterol levels to rise and definitely contributes to the likelihood of developing coronary heart disease. The good news is that the risk of sudden cardiac death and heart attack begins to decline quite soon after stopping smoking, probably within a month or two. The risk thereafter declines toward a level seen in a "never smoker" probably within five to seven years of quitting. It is therefore very important to emphasize that it is never too late to stop smoking. You will, of course, not need to be reminded that there are a great many health hazards to smoking other than causing coronary heart disease and sudden death, including lung cancer and many other cancers, chronic bronchitis, premature aging, and the psychological costs of nicotine addiction.

How do you stop smoking?

We do not intend to give a detailed description of all of the methods to help smokers kick the habit. Any of these, including "stopping cold turkey" (which can be surprisingly effective for many), using nicotine substitutes such as gum or patches, hypnosis, a[illegible]puncture, the use of support materials (e.g., tapes and videos), support groups, and yoga or biofeedback, can be helpful for individual patients. The common denominator for all methods of quitting is the desire, the will and the commitment to stop. This requires an active decision on the part of the smoker; and trying to stop smoking because others want you to will generally not result in success. The fact that psychological preparation for quitting is crucial has not been sufficiently emphasized. The same kind of psychological preparation is required as for any other kind of behavior change, including adopting a new dietary habit, beginning a regular exercise program, and so on.

WOMEN AND HEART DISEASE

THE ISSUE OF coronary heart disease in women has received much attention lately. Women are unfortunately not at all immune from heart disease, and in fact heart disease is the most common cause of death in women in Western society. Women do have a lower likelihood of developing heart disease in their middle years, especially before menopause. Over time, however, the chance of developing heart disease in women increases to approach that of men by their eighth decade of life.

Since women are protected from coronary artery disease to a large extent by the presence of female hormones (largely *estrogen*), they tend to be somewhat older than men when they first develop the signs and symptoms of heart disease, and they tend to be more likely to have coexisting illnesses that can contribute to coronary heart disease, especially diabetes (see page 191). For this reason, the typical female patient first develops heart-related problems when she is older; as well, she is more likely to have high blood pressure and diabetes, and to be somewhat sicker than her male counterpart. This reason accounts for most of the apparent differences between men and women who have coronary heart disease, as opposed to some special biology of heart disease in women. Largely because of these differences in underlying disease, women tend to have symptoms that are more often unusual, such as nausea, a generalized feeling of being unwell or breathlessness, rather than *chest pain*, or *discomfort*, and they are likely to have more serious heart disease when first diagnosed. Whether it is because of these factors or because female patients are less attuned to the possibility that they may have heart disease, women do take longer to go to their doctors or to the hospital at the first sign of coronary heart disease symptoms or a heart attack. Although it is controversial whether they are as likely to undergo extensive testing as men, it is important for female patients and their families to be aware of the possibility of heart disease, and to seek medical care promptly if they have unusual symptoms of severe fatigue, breathlessness, chest discomfort or other disabling symptoms, especially if they have a history of high blood pressure or diabetes.

Once a diagnosis of coronary heart disease is made, women are usually treated just as carefully and thoroughly as men, although their prognosis is unfortunately not as good as the average man's; as noted above, this is the case because they are likely to be older and somewhat sicker at the time that the illness first occurs.

The question of whether estrogen, taken in tablet form or through a skin patch, can prevent or protect from the development of heart disease in women after menopause remains unanswered. A considerable body of research suggests that those women who take estrogen are less likely to develop coronary heart disease, heart attacks and premature cardiac death than those who do not. As it is known that estrogen protects blood vessels and protects against hardening of the arteries, it is probable that hormone supplementation will prevent the development or progression of coronary heart disease in most women. However, at the time of this writing, no large independent study has confirmed the benefit of estrogen in this regard; several very large studies are ongoing and their findings should be available in the near future. Until then, the decision of whether or not to take estrogen will be arrived at after a thorough discussion between a woman and her doctor. Important considerations in making this decision are the knowledge that estrogen alleviates some of the symptoms of menopause, such as hot flushes, and retards the development of *osteoporosis*, or "softening of the bones." The risks of hormone replacement are of developing cancer of the lining of the uterus, the *endometrium*, and possibly of developing breast cancer. It is important to note that the lifetime risk of coronary heart disease is far higher than the lifetime risk of breast cancer, even if hormone therapy does increase the risk of cancer somewhat. Because of these complex competing risks, the decision as to whether or not to take estrogen should not be made lightly.

Many rehabilitation programs, at least until recently, have focused on exercise and not emphasized the social and emotional impact of heart disease. Perhaps as a result, fewer women than men have participated in these programs. Since the needs of women patients are often somewhat different from those of men, they can benefit from one of the specialized *women's programs* recently started for women with heart disease. These programs are particularly recommended for those women who do not find traditional cardiac rehabilitation programs practical or accessible.

CHAPTER 10

Mind: Key Emotional Issues for Those with Heart Disease

ANXIETY

ANXIETY IS A FEELING that almost everybody has experienced. It is the feeling of nervousness, of apprehension, of internal shakiness, and it is commonly associated with unpleasant bodily sensations. It is experienced *directly* as fear, if related to a specific feared object, or generally as *anxiety*; an intense form is panic anxiety. In the *thinking* realm, anxiety can be expressed as worry, or disturbance of concentration. It can be felt in the *muscles* of the body as tension or restlessness, or in different *bodily systems*, such as butterflies in the stomach, diarrhea, dizziness, increased urination, and, in the context of this book, as chest pain, palpitations, shortness of breath and sweating.

Anxiety has a normal function—that is, it signals a *threat*. Following a cardiac event, anxiety is common and normal in the early phases, from the lead-up to the event, through the aftermath and especially during emotional reaction, which is characteristic of the early recuperation phase. Anxiety is understandable, given the threat to the person in the recent past and especially in relation to the possibility of another event occurring. As recuperation becomes well established, anxiety will tend to settle down. This is closely related to the subsidence of physical symptoms. This brings us to a common problem pattern, shown in Figure 10.1.

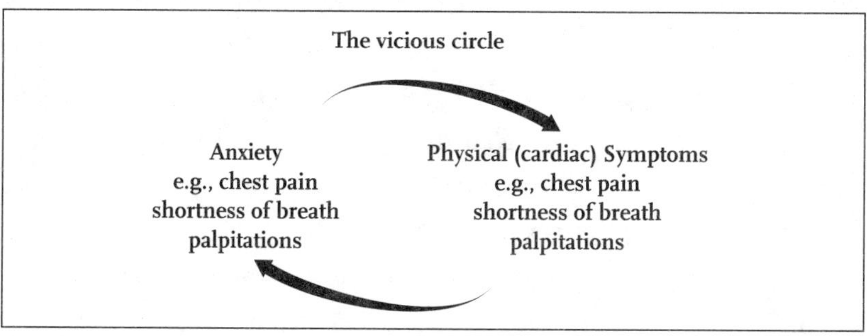

Fig. 10.1

In the early recuperation phase, the patient is typically going through emotional reaction, but, at the same time, physical symptoms, such as chest pain, palpitations, fatigue and shortness of breath, can be fairly prominent. As you will already have noticed, these are the same as, or very similar to, symptoms of anxiety. How is the individual to know which is which? Furthermore, as symptoms such as chest pain can represent a threat to the person, this, in itself, induces anxiety. With more anxiety comes more symptoms, and, presto!—a vicious circle is born.

At this point, we must mention two forms of anxiety that are common, and contribute to this scenario. We emphasize that we are referring to a situation where the cardiologist has reassured the patient that the particular symptom does not pose a danger. The first form of anxiety, which some people experience more strongly than do others, is a tendency to worry excessively or, in fact, to become convinced that a serious medical event is going to occur. This is the only context in which the adjective "hypochondriacal" should be used. As we explained in Part One, "The Guide," it is quite understandable that a symptomatic person who has had a cardiac event might become overly concerned, but some do to excess.

The second case is that of pronounced bodily symptoms (such as palpitations, breathlessness, dizziness) in individuals with heart disease who are found to have a manifestation of panic anxiety or panic disorder. It must be made clear that, for these patients, panic itself does not have to be felt! It seems strange, but we are learning that what we call panic attacks can be expressed by the body alone, causing intense symptoms that the doctors often dismiss; but they are signs that there *is* something wrong. This situation is regrettable, because panic disorder is very treatable.

So, to reiterate, we have described the situation of a vicious circle of bodily symptoms and anxiety that often occur in the post-CAD patient, and which can occur more prominently in the case of persons with a hypochondriacal tendency and in those who are actually suffering panic attacks. However, these patients can also develop further heart problems, and need regular monitoring. If there is change in symptoms, they need to be reevaluated. We all know that even hypochondriacal patients can get ill!

In cases of normal anxiety, we expect a fluctuation and improvement over time. This is helped by being aware, and being able to reassure oneself, of the journey from event to recovery. It is one of the cardinal signs of rehabilitation, that emotional symptoms subside and are replaced by the upbeat tide of reconstruction. So, if the anxiety does not subside, but persists—and, obviously, if it worsens or becomes intolerable at any time—you will need to consult a health-care professional. We will leave it to that person to determine what it is that is troubling you. Usually, such patients will have visited their doctors more often than others, and examination for complicating medical conditions will have been performed; in any case, medical evaluation must be obtained.

If the patient is deemed to be anxious, there are many strategies that can help. It is always important that the physician take the person seriously, in the sense of not dismissing the patient's complaints as "not real." If repeated visits have been a problem in the case of a truly hypochondriacal response, it is helpful to set up regular appointments with the doctor where concerns can be addressed and psychotherapy can be given.

If the patient is found to have panic anxiety, true panic attacks or panic disorder, there is more specific treatment given and the professional can be consulted about this.

For all patients, relaxation techniques are recommended. These are described below, but we are asking that they be formally taught, individually or in the group setting. In the case of a person who has prominent anxiety, we recommend an individualized approach. "Psychotherapy" refers to any "talking treatment." There will always be contexts in which the anxiety occurs, and an experienced psychotherapist can help to work through any problems that are associated with particular situations. Many patients are given tranquilizers in the hospital, and they request them when they are anxious on arrival home. The problem with these medications is twofold—they can lose their effectiveness, and, if not, you have to keep taking them. If you suddenly stop tranquilizers, which you should *not* do, withdrawal effects can occur. A similar situation occurs with sleeping tablets, which are often in the same tranquilizer family. Medication may well be needed in the case of panic disorder, and this can be discussed more fully with your physician.

For anxiety that is well established and for panic disorder, a more rigorous type of psychotherapy, cognitive therapy (or cognitive behavior therapy, if there are associated behavioral issues), can be used. We will soon understand more clearly how patients recovering from a cardiac event will respond to such therapy, but it is likely that, in the future, modified forms of targeted cognitive therapy may be appropriate for such patients with mild panic disorder.

For most people, the anxiety will subside after a cardiac event and reassurance will be sufficient. What you should then do will depend on the progress that you have made, and also on your "vulnerability." There is good evidence that relaxation techniques can be helpful whatever your mood state, and we recommend them across the board; there are also other approaches to what you can do to deal with stress and help improve your CAD outcome. There is much overlap of techniques for the vulnerabilities, and we ask that you review the section "Stress management and the seven vulnerabilities" (pages 219–236) to see what is relevant for you.

Significant others, especially those closest to the patient, can naturally also experience the same type of anxiety as the patient, and may similarly require management, either self-taught or, if symptoms are prominent, more formal.

DEPRESSION

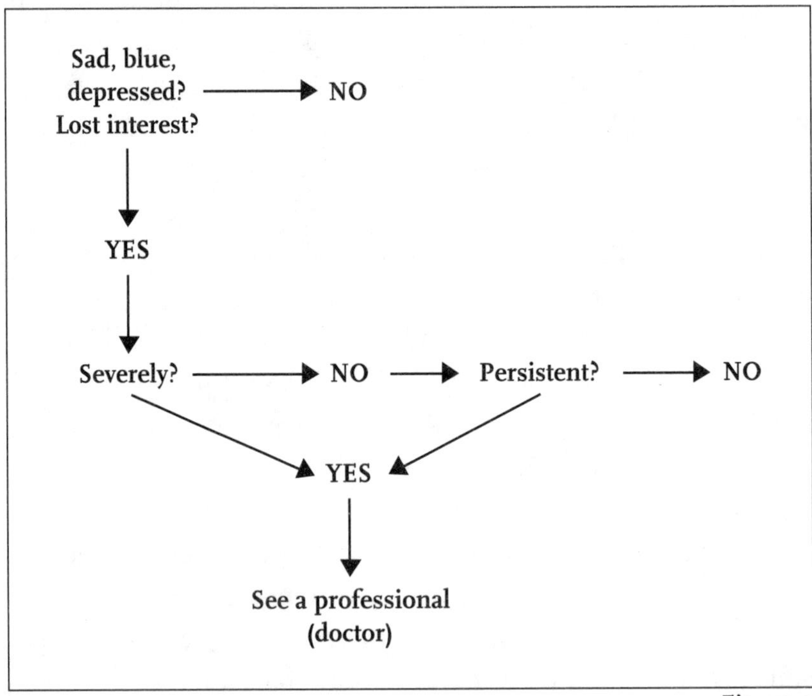

Fig. 10.2

Are you depressed?

Are you feeling sad, blue or depressed?
Have you lost interest or pleasure in your activities?

If your answer is NO to both of these questions, then you are probably reading this for information purposes only, or you may have experienced low mood at another time. You may proceed to the next section ("Clinical Depression").

We now ask: ***Do you feel so bad that you cannot cope? So negative that you feel desperate? That life is not worth living?***

If your answer is YES to any of these questions, then we must abandon our series of queries to ask you to arrange to be assessed by your professional, usually your family doctor or psychiatrist.

If your answer is NO, then proceed with the next two questions:

Have your feelings of sadness, lack of interest or depression gone on for most of the time for* more than two weeks*?

You may also have changes in appetite, sleep disturbances, feeling tired or weak, poor concentration, feeling worthless or have had thoughts about death.

If you answered YES, you *need to be evaluated* by a professional—your family doctor or psychiatrist.

If your complaint becomes severe or continuous, we *also recommend* that you be assessed by your professional. Otherwise, those of you who answered NO to these questions are likely going through, or have gone through, a normal response to the cardiac event, as we explained in Chapter 5. If you experience depressive symptoms (as above) *in the future*, please see below and consult your doctor.

First, we need to *rule out* a clinical depression. Second, we want to alert those who *may become* clinically depressed. Third, we want to *monitor* those whose symptoms are not severe, but continue over time, and could probably benefit from some time of intervention. This third group has what we call "persistent low mood."

Clinical depression

It is important to identify clinical depression for the present and for the future; for what it does to your emotional as well as your physical state.

In the *present*, depression means you are "pressed down," you are unhappy and have poor quality of life. It is hard to conduct your life as you struggle with the "cloud," the "beast" or whatever metaphor you wish to use. Your life is disrupted. Usually, you don't know what is happening to you, and the way you deal with your experience can further complicate the situation, for example, if you blame yourself.

For the *future*, depression, if untreated, means the establishment of a pattern that continues over time. In some cases, depression can be related to self-destruction, even to ending one's life. For most, it simply means an ongoing pattern of poor quality of life that can take many months to get over.

Clinical depression and CAD

The relation of depression to CAD is starting to become clear. We need to take note of the overlap between symptoms of depression and the consequences of the cardiac event, such as fatigue and low motivation. The symptoms of depression retard the healing process after a cardiac event, especially if the depression is not identified and treated. Many depressed patients are mistakenly labeled as "noncompliant," whereas they are apparently unable to be compliant for good reason—they are depressed.

We have mentioned the link between depression and CAD outcome following an event like heart attack (see Chapter 5). Research suggests that those with depression are more liable to die in the six months following a heart attack than are the nondepressed. These studies are not very large, but the finding is consistent. We do not fully understand the mechanism behind the connection between clinical depression and cardiac outcome; this is still being studied, and the link with outcome is less clear, especially for those who have *not* had a heart attack but have had other cardiac events.

Evaluation and treatment of clinical depression

We have purposely not gone into details about the diagnosis of clinical depression, as this must be done by a *professional.* We will make a few general points, though, which we feel to be relevant to those who have been diagnosed as clinically depressed and who also are recovering from a cardiac event.

The first point is that clinical depression is very treatable, but must be handled by a professional, such as a family doctor or psychiatrist or clinical psychologist. Treatment will take place over months, will include close monitoring of the patient and will always consist of some type of talking therapy (psychotherapy). Commonly, antidepressant medication is used as well. When clinical depression is mild, there is accumulating evidence that a type of psychotherapy called "cognitive therapy" can be effective.

As opposed to the older types of antidepressants, the newer medications have shown themselves to be much more heart-friendly, since the release of fluoxetine (or Prozac) about ten years ago. However, this does not mean that side effects or interactions don't occur.

We are still cautious in the early period after heart attack. We recommend that, before a patient who has had a cardiac event is started on antidepressants, his or her cardiologist be informed.

Initial success rate for each antidepressant is about 70 percent; once the correct medication has been identified the rate rises to include almost all patients. The medications invariably take about four weeks to work, and in the early stages can give rise to side effects. These mostly subside, but, if they are prominent, use of the particular antidepressant should be suspended until the situation is discussed with the doctor. In any case, monitoring will be done within a couple of weeks after diagnosis, and then will depend on how the patient is doing. These days, the policy is usually to keep patients on antidepressants for at least six months.

Clinical depression is felt to be linked to a disturbance of brain chemistry, along with *negative patterns of thinking* that become established. It is these patterns ("stinking thinking," as someone put it) that cognitive therapy focuses on. The effectiveness of cognitive therapy for depressed patients after cardiac events is still being evaluated; so far, results appear encouraging. However, patients must be aware that cognitive therapy requires them to do therapy *work*, that is, extra effort between sessions, which is not something that the moderately or severely depressed patients, especially in the throes of their recovery after a cardiac event, may be ready for. However, for the motivated person who is mildly clinically depressed, and for those with persistent low mood, cognitive therapy could well become a treatment of choice in the cardiac patient.

Persistent low mood

Not only are the clinically depressed at risk for poorer outcome after heart attack, but those with persistent low mood—those who have been down or felt blue on an *ongoing* basis—have also been found to be vulnerable. For those with CAD and persistent low mood who have not had a heart attack, the evidence is still being examined. We know, for example, that about one out of six patients develop clinical depression following a heart attack and, in addition, a further one-sixth of the heart-attack group has persistent low mood. Patients are probably unaware that the way they experience their lives, by feeling somewhat down on an ongoing basis, is abnormal. But, like clinical depression, persistent low mood is bad not only for your quality of life, but also for your outcome after a cardiac event. Persistent low mood is probably related to more noncompliance in treatment after a cardiac event, and this may, in part, account for the negative effect on CAD outcome.

Patients with persistent low mood will often have had a history of low mood over the course of their lives. Whether there is an underlying biochemical disturbance, as with clinical depression, remains to be determined; it seems very likely, though, that the psychological components, such as a history of negative thinking patterns, are prominent. It is for this reason, as well as the relative mildness of the condition (as opposed to moderate or severe clinical depression) that makes persistent low mood ideal for interventions such as cognitive therapy. Researchers are currently investigating whether group or abbreviated cognitive approaches, such as learning from educational materials, can be effective in the CAD population with persistent low mood.

For those of you who have had low mood, including sadness or negative thinking, that does not subside, an evaluation is recommended. Initially, a doctor should be consulted; thereafter, if thought necessary, you can be referred for the appropriate therapy.

STRESS AND CAD

ARE STRESS AND HEART attack connected? Most people take this link for granted. A brief review of this question will show that, like most things, this is a complex issue. (The answer, incidentally, is: yes and no!)

First of all, what is "stress"? The trouble is that the meaning of the term has become so diluted over time that there is little left of substance. We will take a loose definition for the moment and refer to stress as "demands which are placed on us or events that are demanding to us." The first realization is that *stress is part of life*—it is in the nature of things. This seemingly obvious statement actually contains much wisdom. M. Scott Peck demonstrated this in his elegantly written *The Road Less Traveled*, whose essential message is that "life is hard": stress is normal; learn to deal with it! This message is important for readers of this book as well: on our journey, stress is predictable, so we need not be taken aback when stress occurs. If we learn to deal with stress, we can take pride in the mastery and maybe even thrill to the challenge. (There is even a book titled *The Joy of Stress*!)

But stress can be excessive. In this book, we have emphasized the "normal" response to a stressful event. However, in the course of life, we all experience events that undoubtedly have impact on us. Interestingly, events that are obviously stressful in an unpleasant way (such as the death of a loved one) and also those that are positive and exciting (such as getting married) have been found to be *stressors* (that is, to cause stress). However, the *reaction* to the stress (what is often called "distress") rather than the stress itself is what determines its health impact. This may explain why patients who have lives that are more "stressful"—busier, more varied and more demanding—may not have higher rates of heart disease than those whose lives are less demanding but not satisfying or subjectively difficult for them.

Another type of stress is *ongoing* demands placed on us. The obvious example here is that of the work setting. It has been found that, when the level of work is heavy (working hard and fast) and the control is limited ("you must do it by a certain time"), the result is stress on the cardiovascular system. But demands are part of work, otherwise they wouldn't pay us to do it! This brings us to the question of how we feel the stress, or our "distress." Each individual processes stress differently, and so feels the effects differently. There is some controversy about the link between emotional stress and cardiac events. How can we say that it was the distress that caused the cardiac event? When researchers find emotional upset before such events, this finding is contaminated by the bias of what you remember and the fact that you have had a heart attack in between! Furthermore, distress is not an isolated phenomenon for any of us. A famous case is that of the surgeon John Hunter, always described as irascible (easy to anger) and aware of it, who in 1793 expired after a particular angry exchange. But if Mr. Hunter was always tending towards irascibility, and died after one episode, how can we honestly say that this proves causality? It is possible that persistent anger and hot-temperedness aggravate a cardiovascular tendency to having a cardiac event (say, a heart attack). The anger episode can then be seen as a *precipitating factor*, or trigger; but a trigger is different from a cause. What we are saying is that emotional factors may well affect cardiovascular disease and trigger cardiac events in the presence of CAD, but that emotional events causing CAD can be seen as rare. Of course, learning about triggers is important, so that if we have the unhealthy tendencies we can try to adjust them.

We now do not focus on Type A personality *per se* because the research has not consistently proven it to confer a risk for CAD.

However, while the evidence for the link with CAD is questioned by recent research, more promising is the isolation of *components* of Type A that seem more directly related to cardiac outcome. The main component is anger or hostility. While still inconclusive, it appears that ongoing thoughts, feelings and behavior (alone or in combination) that are angry, cynical or hostile may confer a risk for cardiac events. Redford Williams and Virginia Williams's book *Anger Kills* discusses this association and what to do about it. We have already said that anger is a normal transient reaction to a cardiac event.

Time pressure is another component of Type A and, for the longest time, has been associated with cardiac patients. Research has not directly linked this to cardiac outcome, but such patients are regularly seen in clinical and research practice and they can also benefit from learning stress-management techniques, especially the time-management component. An ongoing tendency to anxiety—and this includes worrying about having another cardiac event or dying—is also regarded as something to be dealt with, not only because it may aggravate CAD outcome, but especially because it greatly influences one's quality of life. Persons who have been termed "hot reactors" are those who develop a fast heart rate and increased blood pressure or who get flushed with even minor stress and may also benefit from stress-management programs (see Chapter 9).

What is finally emerging in the research literature is the importance of spirituality to our lives and to cardiac outcome. It is hard to disentangle other factors, such as social support, but the belief component appears to be the key ingredient. Dr Erik Erikson always emphasized the substantial role that trust plays in our dealing with the world and the people in it (see his *Childhood and Society*). Trust is important in our interpersonal relationships, but a broad-based belief in the order and meaning of life helps us to deal with the vicissitudes (ups and downs) in the journey of life, including CAD.

Social support has been found to be a consistent protective factor for CAD. Research is still trying to narrow down what this means. Unfortunately, research has a habit of "overfocusing"—it's like trying to look at something small; we cannot see it until we look into the microscope, but then with greater magnification the picture is blurred again! We don't know if the best measure is how you perceive the support you get, the actual supportive relationships or the number of supporting people in your social network. In organized religion and in the rehabilitation programs, we also see the importance of the social support component. Whatever aspect it is, and it may be different ones for different people, we know that social support is good for you, and probably helps improve your cardiac outcome.

STRESS MANAGEMENT AND THE SEVEN VULNERABILITIES

WE USE THE TERM "stress" to denote the *demands* of life, which, as we have repeatedly pointed out, are part of life and cannot be completely avoided. The first step is for you to *identify* the stressors—the *causes* of stress—in your life. We will assume that the cardiac event itself, and the consequences of it, are prominent stressors for you. And, although we do not know you, we do have a fair idea of what types of stress you may encounter. Within the contexts of daily life—and particularly the common ones of home and work—are areas of greatest significance to most people. These include the marital relationship, other close relationships, one's health, work and finances; other areas, such as religion and the social and political situation may also have profound effects on us. We also look to the activities of daily life, the infrastructure that carries us along, and the typical things that happen to provide hassles, stress and, occasionally, trauma.

While stress can be seen as the demands that are placed on us, the other source of stress is what is *removed* from us. We can use one all-embracing theory to explain this other source of stress. There is one force that binds us through life—what John Bowlby has called "attachment." It is the quality of our attachments that will determine, in part, how we will cope when we are *threatened* by the breaking of the attachment—or separation—and the ultimate occurs—that is, *loss.* For convenience, we can look again at those five areas that we mentioned as those of greatest significance—the primary (usually marital) and other close relationships, health, work and finances—and we can see why demands and loss are the key stressors in our lives.

So, we have identified the stressors, and the common *context* of those stressors, and this will greatly help us to begin to deal with stress. Next, we need to closely examine the patterns of our lives and the patterns of our stress. If we have had a series of unpleasant events occur, we cannot go by that track record alone. Many people operate under the assumption that a black cloud hovers overhead and always rains on *them*. There is some reason to believe that having such an attitude in some way predisposes people to keep having more things happen to them. Because pessimists focus on the negative, they are able to convince themselves that worse things are happening to *them*, as compared to the rest of us.

The next thing we need to do is to identify *how we manage stress*. Do we deal with it with no problem? Or, as most will contend, it is only when it gets excessive that the problems start. But what is excessive for some may be no problem for others. The negative feelings we get with stress—*distress*—may be experienced directly, as an unpleasant emotional state, or may be translated into other forms: emotionally, as anxiety or depression, or converted into bodily complaints based on the various bodily systems such as cardiovascular (chest pain, palpitations) or gastrointestinal (diarrhea, nervous stomach).

To sum up: We need to identify both the stress and the distress in our lives, to start to formulate what, in fact, is going on, so that we can best deal with it.

We approach the question of stress management for the patient with CAD by highlighting seven areas of vulnerability, and by giving guidelines for how to deal with these areas. We are using seven "types" to serve as reminders, and we give them names, with apologies to the fairy-tale dwarfs.

1. Heavy: Dealing with stress overload

Before we discuss areas of vulnerability *within* the self, we need to look *without.* The first thing that is directly affecting us is the fact of a recent cardiac event, which has such an impact that it can take up to a year or more to achieve recovery. With this in mind, we must be aware of the vulnerable state that we are in, in terms of having extra stress in our lives. At the same time, our own lives, and the lives of those to whom we are tied, inexorably go on, and there is the natural ebb and flow of demands and the lack thereof, of hard times and easy times. We must be aware of the stressors in our lives, since, especially during this vulnerable time of the recovery process, *we should not overload ourselves.* The demand or load can be too "heavy."

As you recover from the cardiac event, your level of stress tolerance is going to increase. This is particularly the case once you are well into the rehabilitation phase. At first it is important that no *extra* avoidable stressors be added, so that each person can have the benefit of all the positive aspects of this phase. A basic tenet of this book is that of *timing.* Of course, when it comes to stress it is not always possible to defer or avoid it. But if you are on your toes, and by this we mean more aware of stress and your reaction to it, you will know *when* you are best able to deal with whatever is handed to you. If you are in a particularly vulnerable period, say, in the aftermath or early recuperation phase, you will have a good excuse to try to defer a particular stressor.

Though we may well return to our own vulnerabilities and issues that create the environment in which too much stress accumulates (such as with overaccommodating behavior, see "Softy"), we should, first of all, determine whether there is too much stress in our lives. The problem here is usually one of context. We may enter into a situation, be it in the home or at work, where on an ongoing basis there is too much demand. The load may be too great, or there may be a problem of time pressure. This particularly occurs at work, where deadlines are prominent. The notion of "job strain" has been defined as too much job demand and too little control. At home, overly submissive spouses may find themselves doing more than their fair share, particularly when it comes to the rearing of the children and the running of the house. A situation of overload is liable to occur when a person is already vulnerable, by virtue of having another ongoing problem. This is where having recently gone through a cardiac event, and then having to deal with *further* demands, may prove too stressful for some. Again, we have a wide variation within what some can do quite easily and what others struggle with.

So, you need to *become aware of your stress load.* If we take the common context of work and the notion of avoiding stress overload, but keep in mind that the demands of work are what we are being paid for and seem duty-bound to accept, invariably we are talking about a graded approach to returning to work after a cardiac event. Not all stress at work is obligatory. If you analyze it, you may well find that you are taking too much on because of your tendency to agree with what others ask you to do. This is not surprising, especially if those people are your boss and supervisors! We will be discussing in greater detail the question of *allowing* too much. There are diplomatic ways of dealing with these issues. We are referring to the notion of *assertiveness*, a focused and practical way of dealing with these issues (see "Softy"). If practical, try to take on less work that contributes to work overload, delegating or sharing or declining diplomatically whenever possible. For what we must do, apportion the time component, and pace the work so that there will be no period of time, such as just before deadlines, when we are truly weighed down by work. Remember that preparedness is half the job and that, if we think on our feet, we can avoid most overload situations.

2. Edgy and Shaky: Relaxation techniques

We are addressing this to all those patients who are subject to anxiety, being "hyper" or overstimulated (in the sense of being "on the alert") for much of the time. There is inconclusive evidence that this type of person may be at risk for more cardiac events than others, based on the theory that the cardiovascular system is set at a pitch that is unhealthy to sustain, much in the same way that an engine idles too high; increase the pressure and you will be in the red zone. It may also relate to those who have a concomitant cardiovascular response. By this we mean that with stress, the heart rate or blood pressure rapidly increases, and flushing may occur, but this subsides with the passage of the stress. The "edginess" we describe in this section can spill over into other vulnerabilities highlighted in the other sections; so don't be surprised if you identify with the other tendencies. In particular, we see a cluster of those who identify with this section (Edgy), together with Angry, Pushy, Busy and Hurry. So, don't be surprised if they all seem to merge together; they do, because they go together.

We are also addressing those who read about and identified with anxiety and related symptoms in this book. To both, we are prepared to make a broad-based recommendation about relaxation techniques: they can benefit almost anybody, and one day they may be included in general rehabilitation programs, in the same way that exercise is routinely included nowadays. Are we getting carried away? We think so, to a certain extent, but as a counterpart to the "burn-off" of exercise, there is the "calm-down" of relaxation techniques. They are starting to enter the mainstream as approaches to dealing with CAD and all other types of illness, such as cancer, and are being incorporated into wellness programs everywhere. A boost was supplied in the 1970s with the publication of *The Relaxation Response* by Herbert Benson. In it, he describes a simple method for evoking the physiological as well as the psychological response of relaxation. The technique involved just two basic components: focusing and defocusing.

Defocusing involves shutting out of your consciousness all the thoughts and feelings—the "distracting noises"—that enter your mind as a matter of course. For those of you who are Edgy or Shaky, this will be more easily said than done, as you are the type of person whose thoughts and feelings seem irresistibly impelled into your minds. You will need to learn to push these intrusions away. There is a fine art in doing this; you will find that if you try too hard, you may create a boomerang effect. We are talking about a gentle easing away, rather than a forceful pushing aside.

Ideally, we recommend that you actively seek training in the *focusing* techniques. Just reading about them may get you into bad habits that are not easily corrected. So, you need to find someone with expertise in relaxation training. Should you learn individually or in a group setting? If you do not have prominent symptoms and a group is recommended by professionals or by fellow CAD patients, please go ahead; otherwise, we suggest an individualized program, which includes evaluation and learning of the basic techniques, one of which is taught each week; you will be able to demonstrate your ability to master each technique. The relaxation techniques are: deep breathing, progressive muscular relaxation, autogenic relaxation, imaging and meditation. *Deep breathing* is controlled, slow and deep, and has an abdominal component. *Progressive muscular relaxation* is familiar to many who have gone through prenatal classes, including the husbands! It is most effective as an initiator of a relaxation sequence; however, in a tense or "hyper" person it can be used with effect, and unnoticeably, for relaxation of the muscles. With *autogenic relaxation*, your mind focuses on specific muscle groups in terms of how they feel—hot or heavy, for example. *Imaging* is a skill well worth having; it involves conjuring up in the mind a scene that is full of relaxing cues, such as lying on a beach in Tahiti, with the waves lapping on the shore as the sun beats down. Although the relaxation therapist in the group setting will suggest a specific scene, in the end each individual will need to conjure up his or her own relaxing scene, as what makes *you* relaxed can have the opposite effect on someone else. We recommend imaging (imagining a relaxing scene) rather than active visualization (where an empowering story, such as fighting heart disease, is fantasized). *Meditation* can be the most difficult, but, in the end, the most satisfying of the relaxation techniques. This is particularly so if you see yourself as Mr. or Ms. Busy (see below), and are uncomfortable when your mind is not occupied. Being defocused is difficult for you, but once you persist with the meditation technique, your symptoms should subside, and soon you will develop the expertise to produce the relaxation response on demand.

At the end of the relaxation course, you will become familiar with what works for you. You should then start to practice these techniques with the same frequency as a maintenance exercise program, that is, at least four times a week. The sequence is devised specifically for you, and usually consists of three of the techniques (for example, starting with progressive muscular relaxation, going on to deep breathing, and ending with meditation). The techniques should become second nature to you so that you can apply them in your daily life when you become anxious, "hyper," tense, or whatever is responsive to the techniques.

3. Angry and Pushy: Anger management

Anger is part of the human condition. If we are provoked, threatened or frustrated, it will emerge, as a "slow burn," a flare-up or an explosion. We deal here with two aspects of anger; the first relates to anger as part of the response to a cardiac event; the second, to an ongoing emotional pattern.

The outcry "Why me?" epitomizes the anger that typically occurs during the emotional reaction of recuperation (see Chapter 5). This emotional response will naturally subside over time, depending on what actually happens medically during recovery. As we expect it to subside, there is no need to have special treatment for the anger, unless it persists over time. It is uncommon for this to occur when there is no history of anger. Researchers are starting to discover what personality "type" is predisposed to be "Angry." These people tend to be cynical about the world; they have an underlying sense of mistrust, and they attribute bad intent to other people.

Many of our readers will be familiar with the term "Type A personality." A number of years ago evidence was found to show that Type A was associated with an increased risk of CAD and worse outcome in CAD patients. However, as the years went on, subsequent studies failed to convincingly show that this was the case, despite the fact that the three components of Type A behavior—anger, time urgency and competitive behavior patterns—are commonly found in CAD patients. What now emerges on reanalysis of the data is that one of the three components, anger or hostility, does show a fairly consistent relationship with CAD outcome.

"Pushy" is associated with two related characteristics: aggression and competitiveness. "Aggression" refers not only to the feeling of anger, but also to how you conduct yourself in your dealings with people at home, in your career and in your life generally. You are competitive, achievement-driven and "striving"—a restless soul on the horizontal escalator of life. "Achievement" usually refers to how well you do in the work setting, but a closer look shows us that it permeates most aspects, from status in your social structure, to family and ultimately to self-esteem. In sum, the "pushy" need to drive themselves to achieve, and this trait has been noted with CAD patients. We are not convinced that these characteristics are necessarily found in more abundance in CAD patients, but when such individuals already have a tendency to CAD, then these characteristics may have a negative impact on cardiac outcome.

Pushy patients with these personality characteristics may have more trouble dealing with recuperation, but may do well with rehabilitation. However, in the long term, if aggression and competitiveness are prominent, attempting to tone them down is a heart-healthy alternative.

In light of the research findings linking anger with CAD outcome, efforts have been made to reduce anger in CAD patients in order to potentially improve their cardiac outcome. We first need to see what we are trying to change before specific treatments are offered. We take into consideration whether the patient has suffered a recent cardiac event, in which case listening, understanding and support may be all that is necessary. However, should the feelings, thoughts, and especially the expression of anger continue into the rehabilitation phase, consideration should be given to doing an anger-management program. Invariably this will be combined with relaxation training, as anger so commonly occurs in the context of high arousal. Another way of putting this is to see anger as being the other side of the "fight or flight" mechanism, which programs animals and humans to deal with the threats they encounter. Anger management can be learned individually, but this is one program that can be carried out even more effectively in a group setting.

The theory of anger management is set out very simply in the Williamses' book *Anger Kills*. First, anger needs to be identified, and here there can be great individual variation, from the common frustration we all experience while driving in traffic to something totally specific to ourselves. Once it is labeled, the angry person asks: Is my continued anger justified? It usually isn't, and then suppression is counseled, but this is difficult, as anger occurs so quickly and strongly. If the anger is justified, then assertiveness is counseled (see "Softy"). The learning of assertiveness skills is particularly helpful and straightforward, and the group setting is invaluable in allowing you to practice what is an interpersonal skill. You can see results quickly, but behaviors need to be reinforced and practiced to sustain good results.

As radical methods are acquired to deal with what is often a fulminant response, researchers have tried to deal with ways of "spotting the cues" or identifying the triggers that set off anger. Each person has his or her own cues, but some are common, such as traffic (road rage) or rude people. While it is relatively easy to identify the cues that set each person off, it can be a Herculean task to turn off or suppress these strong emotions and impulses. A quick, strong counter-response is required, and researchers have gone to great lengths to find methods to deal with this. A reportedly effective method is the "hook," which graphically describes how, like a fish being caught, anger takes over. Patients are taught to shout out the word (or otherwise shout it out silently in their minds) as a short, sharp method to quell the fountain of anger. Groups, which must be run by experienced group leaders, effectively challenge participants, and progress can be made as long as the treatment persists over a period of months. In some cases where anger is hard to contain, particularly if it is associated with low mood and high anxiety, it has been reported that medication can be helpful, but should be administered as an adjunct to the usual anger-management techniques.

The aggressive and competitive individual needs "balance," which we discussed in Chapter 5. Such patients need to reach a point of equilibrium in their home, work and social lives, and particularly in their emotional symptoms. Pacing in terms of how much one does, and balancing in terms of what one does, are basic rules to follow. At the core is the notion of being "centered." In terms of the balance, many are walking a tightrope and can easily fall off. This is understandable soon after a cardiac event, but not on an ongoing basis. Remaining on a solid footing is a goal for all of us, and a challenge for the aggressive and competitive individual.

4. Busy and Hurry: Time management

Rush, rush, rush… Clinicians who treat patients with CAD often encounter the type of individual who has to be doing something. This person is driven by an inner force and must have a focus in life. The big problem occurs when the focus stops. Then, they can experience a deluge of tension, anxiety, negative thoughts, or bodily sensations such as palpitations. These people have to keep moving. In the early phases of aftermath and recuperation, they may bury themselves in activities; unfortunately, doing so is often premature and leads to unfavorable consequences.

The person who solves life's problems through activity often has another characteristic that has long been associated with patients with CAD: the problem of time pressure or time urgency. Psychologists have gone to elaborate extents to describe such behavior. It is not conclusive that this component of Type A confers a negative outcome for CAD patients. However, addressing the issue of time pressure is an important part of treatment and patients feel so much better after they start to slow down. This change involves *pacing*, or control, of activities over time, and adopting relaxation techniques. Exercise is a natural for the time-pressured ("Hurry"); rarely do they need to be told to exercise, as they are very busy exercising already! Relaxation, or the "calm down" approach, is the converse of the "burn-off" approach of exercise, and both can be very useful, although initially, time-pressured people claim they don't "have the time" to learn the relaxation techniques! Meditation is very difficult for them and can lead to a temporary increase of symptoms, but with persistent effort, a general toning down can be achieved. Here it is very important that relaxation be performed routinely, at least four times per week. With time management, the broad area of *self-control* is an underlying theme. The degree to which this can be changed varies among people: for some, it is an adjustment that has to be made; for many, it is a somewhat laborious challenge that becomes more and more resistant to change as the cardiac event recedes into the past. It pays to get into good habits soon; otherwise it is going to be an uphill battle. So, slow down now!

5. Lonely: Why you need the support of others

If we review the research on what emotional factors have an impact on CAD outcome, there is fairly compelling evidence for only three of them. At this time, depression is deservedly grabbing the spotlight. Anger is making an impressive comeback, now that Type A personality is starting to fade as a major risk factor. But a constant finding in the literature is that social support is related to good CAD outcome. Social support usually tends to operate as a "mitigating factor" insofar as cardiac outcome is concerned. That is, unlike depression, and possibly hostility, where the negative effect seems to be a direct one, social support serves to add to or subtract from the other factors that affect outcome.

In terms of social support, it is difficult to define what it is that confers the protection or lack of it in relation to CAD outcome. Are we talking about the socially isolated patient who lacks a social network? Or are we referring to a dearth of social activities that is bad for you? Is it because you may not have enough people who are really close to you, or even one such person? Or, finally, is it simply that you perceive that you are not supported? The answer is probably: some or all of the above! Feeling isolated in the community is a vulnerability factor. Not to have social activities, or generally to have little interaction with others, is probably a type of deprivation, a lack of the nutritious social "food" that most of us seem to require. All therapists—people who spend their time talking to help others deal with emotional issues—will agree that we need not only social contact, but meaningful relationships, most of all. If attachment is what binds us (see Bowlby), then the absence of close relationships is what tears us apart. A term that is often used to describe what we require to feel supported is "confidante," that is, someone to whom we can disclose what we think and feel. If we have even one such person, it will help our emotional and, presumably, our physical health.

But how can we correct the lack of social support? We can't simply go to the local department store and order it. No, this is a challenge for everybody concerned. Most of us just take our social setup for granted. An example is Rose, who is apparently quite content with her friends and her lifestyle, but, during the journey of recovery, places an extra load on her family as she doesn't have close friends to rely on. It is important that we be aware of our social circle, our social activities and, importantly, whether we have any confidantes.

Once we are aware of our social circumstances, we can then appraise what and whom we think is missing in our lives; if we are still not sure, we can discuss this with our loved one or, if there is no such person, a family doctor, social worker or therapist. Occupational therapists seem particularly well trained to review this type of issue and also to provide some solutions.

Social activities are fairly easy to arrange. You simply have to decide what you like to do. The activity should be one that is repeated on a fairly regular basis. This makes it easier to pursue the ulterior motive behind starting such activities: namely, to meet people. You will be doing something you like to do and, in passing, meeting people who, not coincidentally, just happen to have at least one interest in common with you: the specific activity you have chosen. Since meeting people is notoriously a hit-and-miss proposition, you will want to increase your chances of success!

Obviously, it is much easier to revive relationships that are already in place as they have a "track record." However, it is important to examine the issues that accounted for the lapse in the friendship. People are often naïve when it comes to interacting with their fellow humans. We need to remember a basic rule: "Relationships are messy!" If we have a completely conflict-free friendship, the chances are that we have not been too open about our feelings. Disagreement is a normal part of human interaction, and we shouldn't spend our time avoiding it, or we will be unsupported. We need to work through our issues, and so develop meaningful relationships.

6. Touchy: Dealing with the sensitive person

In recent years there has been more interest in the person who is *sensitive* to the world, who finds it difficult to filter out the incoming stimuli of the environment. This individual takes life seriously. He or she is easily upset. Stress, for this person, is not deflected, as it should be; it is *absorbed.* The problem does not end here. With sensitivity comes *reactivity.* The reactive individual often shows a knee-jerk response, and is seemingly unable to do otherwise. We are not talking about a rare bird; sensitive people are everywhere. Probably a portion of the population is so sensitive that they should be aware of this tendency, to avoid hardships in life, particularly if an obvious stressor occurs. Kevin, one of our "Select Six," reacted quite strongly during the early phases after a cardiac event. We showed that he didn't necessarily do worse than the others. Indeed, there seems to be some evidence to show that sensitive subjects, while by definition reacting more strongly, can also derive some benefit from doing so, including a better appreciation of what goes on in the world, both in understanding and, potentially, in the nuances and subtleties of refined pleasure. A better understanding also may allow problems to be solved more quickly and effectively.

On a practical level, sensitive individuals should be aware of this particular tendency and of the likelihood of reacting to stressors. Once such awareness has been achieved, the difficult subject of change must be faced. You will retort that sensitivity is part of your natural self—how in the world can this be changed? You have to accept that this tendency is inherent, but the good news is that it is not completely inflexible. There is room to maneuver. One can learn to shift along the spectrum. Now, we don't want to exaggerate: the movement is slight; however, it is noticeable! So, we can learn to shut out some of the stimuli coming into our lives by focusing on what is consequential for us. Obviously, if it is in our power to avoid what is harmful to us, then we should do so, but we cannot, in good conscience, argue only for avoidance, which can be counterproductive when a problem is faced. But if there is no need to confront a stressor, avoidance is logical. When something occurs and we don't need to take it in, we must start to attempt to screen it out.

The next task is to deal with what we previously thought was irresistible—our reaction. Part of sensitivity is reactivity. The point is that sensitive people tend to overreact. The reaction seems so automatic that many feel it cannot be changed. But, you are able to work on both the intensity and the duration of response. You can reduce how strongly you react, and for how long. You do this by the old-fashioned technique of self-control. We acknowledge that this is not easy, but it can be done. And, the *sooner* you exert the control, the better your chance of success. Once you succeed, you will be inclined to repeat what you have done. To be *really* successful, follow our mantra: practice, practice!

If what occurred to trigger your reaction needs to be dealt with, you can channel your energies into solving the problem. One method—assertiveness—we discuss below. Treatment for the sensitive person is still in its infancy, but if you understand the tendency in yourself and you learn the skills we recommend to strengthen yourself, you can manage your stress more effectively.

7. Softy: Assertiveness

A final area of vulnerability has to do with the way you deal with the demands of life, in particular how you resolve issues with others. When you are asked to do something, do you tend to agree to do it? What happens when you don't want to do something? Will you say so? If the other person is insistent, will you go along with it? Will you fight for your rights? One of the big problems for many people turns out to be that they simply accede more than they should to the demands of others. When it comes to who will prevail, the answer is: the other person. When it comes to who will yield, the answer is: you!

We can broadly define three types of people—those who get their own way, those who negotiate the issues and those who tend to give in to others' demands. Another set of labels—which is convenient, though often inaccurate—aggressive, assertive and accommodating.

Both the aggressive and the accommodating person are, by definition, unassertive. Aggressive people obtain what they want by brute insistence; accommodaters allow aggressors to get what they want. A perfect match, in an imperfect sort of way. Interestingly, if you push one of these types long or hard enough, the other one can emerge. For example, the person who has submitted for too long can snap, and—presto!—out pops aggression. Both "Pushy" and "Softy" can be affected by the recovery process, and their adjustment will be just that much more difficult. But it is also the long-term CAD outcome that we are addressing here. Anger and aggression have been found to be associated with poorer CAD outcome. Is this also the case for submissiveness? This we do not yet know, but as Softy more easily accepts stress, so he or she will consequently be more easily affected by others and may suffer more as a result. The accommodater does not particularly enjoy being overloaded with stress; it is just that he or she doesn't know how to say "no"! For many, this response is so automatic that they don't even realize that they have any options! It must be conceded that in some situations it is genuinely difficult and politically inadvisable to resist a demand or stand up for your rights; say, for example, your boss is your opponent! However, if you are diplomatic and use certain skills, you can often reach a compromise. The skills that we recommend can be learned through assertiveness training.

For the aggressive person, it is important to realize that anger, especially if expressed outwards, has negative effects. People are usually responding to aggression, which is by nature provocative, and so it is common for chain reactions to occur, as people get offended, which in turn offends you, and so on. But, even more important, anger is bad for your health. We mentioned the flowchart in the Williamses's book *Anger Kills*, where this question is asked: Is my continued anger justified? If the answer is no, then the difficult-to-do suppression is advised. However, if the anger is justified, the fine art of *assertiveness* is advised.

Assertiveness is a controlled disposition. It is not emotional, like aggression. It does not yield, like submissiveness. It does not give out the "bad stuff," like the former, or take it in, like the latter. For the Softy, too much "taking in" leads to negativity within the self. Assertiveness allows the "bad stuff" to be deflected, but it uses a logical approach. It takes a stand. It uses negotiation. Assertiveness needs to be formally taught, and we have found the group setting to be very effective, as long as it is run by an experienced group leader.

Assertiveness training is primarily a skills-based approach that uses well-tried simple techniques that include role-playing and limited disclosure. (The book *When I Say No I Feel Guilty* is popular and, while not specifically tailored for CAD patients, it is a useful introduction to the subject.) Group settings are most productive when they include both aggressive and submissive people; this enhances the chemistry! But the truth is that the hidden side of each person will usually be revealed: the soft side of the aggressor, and the angry side of the accommodater.

Groups are not curative. They help in a short, sharp way; but repeated reminders are necessary, and so refresher courses are recommended in the long term. If you practice, assertiveness is something you "always have," and it can help in the other journeys to come.

STRESS AND HEART DISEASE: A PATIENT'S PERSONAL VIEW

THE FOLLOWING WAS written by a patient and represents his own view of what he calls "Heart and Mind."

I sat on the edge of my bed, numb with shock.

Sleep was an eternity away.

Bathed in cold sweat, I struggled for control, breathing in, out, in, out, as slowly and deeply as I could.

Over and over I recited the Twenty-third Psalm: "The Lord is my Shepherd, I shall not want." I read randomly from the psalms of David, responding to whatever words and phrases might keep me from falling into an abyss of seeming insanity.

I seemed to be clinging to life and sanity through absolute faith in a Higher Power above this terrible crisis so vividly happening to me.

The end of that business day, hours before, seemed a lifetime away.

I thought of the three decades of loyalty and discipline, energy and perseverance, color and brilliance in a career that had made me famous and loved in an industry known for its utter competitiveness.

I thought of the company I had helped to found three decades before. How I, more than anyone, had helped to build, and build and rebuild it to a position of leadership and prominence.

I thought of the beloved department I had built—widely acknowledged as the best anywhere in the world.

I thought of all the company's promises of security and rewards.

Of light at the end. The financial means to take care of my family.

Then I recalled the last eighteen months as time got tough, and the top two officers made mistakes, piling on their bad decisions of the last three to four years. They had suddenly taken on seemingly new personalities, striking out like trapped rattlesnakes at almost all around them.

Agonizing harassment. Attempts to breach my integrity. And now this. The breach of my contract with only a few years left to go. And all in a sinister way designed to discredit and destroy my reputation and silently murder my career, casting my body down into a dungeon oubliette.

With no sleep I dressed and arrived downtown at the office of a lawyer I knew to be the best in the business. Fortunately he was there (it was 7.30 A.M).

He began the healing. Throughout the long ordeal I had begun. His reassurance, his gentle kindness, his understanding were a shield and a salvation.

Not many weeks later I sat in my family doctor's office, unaware my blood pressure was 220/120 at rest.

I felt bereaved of my loss of my department (my business family) so much that I cried in the bathtub. For a while I had struggled to quickly rebuild a career elsewhere. My family doctor saved my life (I now believe) by putting me on disability. I had come close to dying of a broken heart.

He made me rest. Gave me psychotherapy. And I began a vigorous program of vegetarian diet, Cooper Aerobics (swimming and walking and treadmill), rest and meditation. I attended several lifestyle sessions in the U.S.A.

About a year after this traumatic episode had shattered my life, I was in for another shock. Despite excellent levels of cholesterol, resting blood pressure at normal, excellent fitness and weight, and several tests that seemed not bad if not totally okay, the results of a nuclear cardiac scan were now in.

My cardiologist, whose life-saving instincts had led him to prescribe this test, informed me that my right coronary artery was probably about 80 percent blocked. I was a candidate for a sudden, no-warning heart attack at any time, with a 30 to 50 percent probability of fatality. (In other words, if the first one didn't kill me, the second or third one would.)

I sat stunned. This had to be happening to somebody else.

I must carry nitroglycerin with me for the rest of my life.

The nuclear pictures showed a heart with severe ischemia, possibly a mild infarction.

Had I suffered a mild heart attack that first night a year ago as I stiffly sweated "cold blood" all that night? Quite possibly so, it was agreed.

I redoubled my lifestyle efforts at healing. Strict adherence to a program of vegetarianism and aerobics, meditation and relaxation, rest and stretching exercises, stress management.

Gradually, after two to three years and several more tests, my nuclear scan moved into a range near normal. But we needed confirmation with another good result over time.

About a year later I awaited the result, fully expecting a normal test. After all, I had stuck to my program year after year.

Then came the next shock. It was the worst scan ever. No blood was going through the right coronary artery at all (no dye = no blood).

How could it be? The doctor asked what was different about my life that last year.

Then I let it all out. I thought, after losing my career and my health, I was now about to lose my wife to cancer. Lumps on the breast. Bad pap tests. Chronic bladder infections. What colossal stress!

The doctors all told me stress, especially mental and emotional stress, was a far more dangerous factor than cholesterol, diet, exercise or anything else.

But the universe was again to be very kind to me. My wife got better. The lumps turned out to be only cysts, the bladder infections finally cleared up and stayed cleared up. The paps became normal. The sunshine of my life was to be with me for a while longer. That stress disappeared.

Eventually, another nuclear test of my heart registered completely normal. The blockage had miraculously gone. The lifestyle program was working after all, as long as I avoided stress.

The frightening thing was that reversibility of artery blockage was clearly two-way. Sensitive to stress, my heart could clear itself over time, then quickly block up under stress, then clear up again when that stress was totally removed.

The focus of my program became centered on stress management. And at this stage of my life (at age sixty and with thirty-five 4,000-hour high-stress business years behind me), stress avoidance. So many of my friends and peers were already dead of heart disease, especially the sudden, no-warning variety to which I was vulnerable. I prayed to avoid their fate. I wished to live.

As the years go by, I see more and more evidence published in the newspapers.

Heart and mind are linked.

Yes, you can literally die of a broken heart.

Stress at work can shoot up a man's blood pressure. Jet cholesterol into his arteries. Produce spasm and blockage.

Sufficiently strong mental stress can clearly override all the other mitigating factors.

I am the living (fortunately living, not dead) proof of that.

This is a "from the heart" outcry from a man after he was let go from work. It is very personal and very emotional. To him, there is no doubt that heart and mind are inextricably linked. We do not wish to debate the actual evidence. Rather, we want to demonstrate in the most vivid way we can—a personal testament to what happened—the actual experience of this link.

We are sure that this patient will admit that he is an emotionally reactive person. He sees his bodily response as a corresponding reaction to the "stress" that he has gone through. He recognizes how "stressed" he had been for all those years, and implies that he had ignored the deleterious effects of those demands; in fact, he may have thrived on them before; now, in his present life, he faces up to what he sees as the toxic effects of the stress; in fact, he sees it as life-threatening. Not surprisingly, from this man's point of view, he must avoid stress, which he studiously does and seems satisfied with his solution.

We acknowledge that this man represents one end of the spectrum; what he experiences may be familiar to only a small number of people. We cannot review here the evidence of the link of heart and mind in his case, but we accept that there is at least some connection. In general, we, as clinicians, do not advocate complete stress avoidance; for one thing, it is not possible! In his case, not working may be an appropriate way to protect his health. But we cannot avoid seeing this man's distress, and if there is evidence of a cardiovascular effect, as there is in some cases, we must work to reduce suffering and the possible bodily consequences.

WHEN TO SEEK COUNSELING, AND FROM WHOM

If urgent	→	emergency department, physician, professional
For all	→	lectures at recommended institutions, discussions at rehab programs
Optional-time-limited	→	educational or support groups or relaxation techniques for patients and spouses
For evaluation	→	family doctor or psychiatrist or psychologist
For family or marital evaluation	→	marital therapist
Individual skills	→	trained professional
Group skills	→	trained professional

Fig. 10.3

We live in strange times for therapy. On the one hand is the undeniable fact that the vast majority of people who require any type of emotional help, from relaxation to drugs, are unattended to; they do not receive any help, or else the help is inadequate. On the other hand, there is the tendency for some people to become "overtherapized." They spend a lot of their time seeking out one treatment after another—"therapy as life." In this book, we are steering a middle ground. We do not ask for people to line up for a succession of psychological treatments. We have already supported the notion of "adaptive denial," whereby it is acceptable to suppress emotional issues as long as the medical treatment is followed. But we must add a caveat: where the emotional issues continue to fester, where the individual remains very much off-center, it will be necessary to confront these issues and restore the emotional balance.

This book is an essay in awareness. By now, you should be much more able to identify what you have gone through, and "where you are at" in your recovery. If you are still in the early phases, say, in the aftermath or recuperation, it will be important to understand that you may well be experiencing a normal emotional reaction to the cardiac event. For many of our readers, time itself will heal. So, when must we proceed to the professional? What can we recommend for everybody?

Let us begin with the identification process. Who is the professional? Everyone will have a general practitioner or family doctor. You must start your quest with this person, who is so important to your well-being. You will have established a trusting patient–doctor relationship, and you will want to check that all the medical aspects have been dealt with; you don't want to receive weeks and months of psychological treatment only to discover that there was a physical basis, say, a cardiac origin or the medication you take, for your present problem.

Some family doctors will have established an interest in treating patients with the type of issues that have arisen since your cardiac event. This may be along the lines of more in-depth counseling, family therapy, or even relaxation training. Otherwise you will be referred to someone who specializes in these particular areas.

At any time, if what you experience is *too much for you to cope with*, say, a severe depression, then you should proceed immediately to your doctor. In an actual emergency, you would go to the emergency room of your local hospital.

So, severity of symptoms is an indicator of your need to leapfrog over the usual decisions that we are going to take you through now, and you must proceed directly to the evaluation-and-treatment option.

Assuming a lack of urgency, who is going to need what? All patients would probably benefit from being aware of the facts, as we now know them, and as we have tried to convey in this book. Lectures and discussions on the emotional aspects of recovery from a cardiac event, in a rehab setting with a trained professional, are recommended. We expect that there will be sessions available to spouses and interested family as well. Review of stress management in this setting is also helpful. In a number of centers, the local Heart Foundation or hospital organization have set up a course of sessions to educate and give support to those recovering from cardiac events; here, again, spouses are usually invited. These courses are time-limited and always run by experienced professionals. The authors support, across the board, the learning of relaxation techniques for regular use, especially for any of the categories of people mentioned above, in the discussion of stress management. For the regular patient, group methods are acceptable, but in cases where symptoms are prominent, we prefer the individualized approach. For other treatment possibilities, we suggest you consult with your family doctor or primary therapist.

Most people who have identified problems in recovery can benefit from specific approaches. For example, problems with anger and assertiveness generally can be referred to the appropriate groups for anger-management and/or assertiveness training. Often there is considerable overlap in these groups, so you should check what specifically is offered.

Support groups for cardiac patients have proliferated. We prefer a time-limited approach, where there is a fixed endpoint to the course of sessions, as compared to an open-ended approach. As well, groups should be moderated by an experienced group leader and clear guidelines for the agenda should be established.

Those patients who require medication for emotional symptoms (such as antidepressants) will need to have access to a physician, and a psychiatrist can be consulted.

If specialized counseling is required, any qualified professional

—psychologist, social worker or one of the doctors mentioned above—can be an acceptable choice; a key question to ask is whether they have experience with cardiac patients. The recommendations of others is, naturally, a pointer for you. Cognitive behavioral therapy requires special expertise; therapists offering it must have been trained in this field. Payment is understandably an issue for many, and this should be clarified prior to the commencement of the course of therapy.

All these recommendations also apply to *the family of the cardiac patient.* Naturally, if the family system itself is not functioning well, the services of an experienced family counselor are required.

PSYCHIATRIC EMERGENCY

AFTER A CARDIAC EVENT, a true psychiatric emergency is uncommon, but, naturally, when it does occur, it is crucial that it be treated. For practical purposes, we describe a sequence of urgency, although it does not necessarily develop in such a systematic way. There may be fleeting thoughts, persistent thoughts, a plan to act and finally the urge to commit suicide. If thoughts of suicide are persistent, a physician should be consulted within the day; if there is any plan or urge to act, proceed to the nearest emergency department. Help is always available, and treatment is effective.

A not uncommon scenario with cardiac patients is the sudden development of acute panic with the fear that one is going to die or lose control or go crazy. This may be accompanied by chest pain, palpitations or other physical symptoms. Patients must be examined by a physician. In the case of cardiac symptoms such as chest pain, cardiac disease must be ruled out—on an emergency basis, if necessary. If cardiac disease as a cause is ruled out, a panic attack is a possibility. There is excellent treatment available for this.

CHAPTER II

Heart to Mind: Three Dialogues between Cardiology and Psychiatry about the Journey of Recovery

"It's a typical modern disease. I think its causes are of a moral order. The great majority of us are required to live a life of constant, systematic duplicity. Your health is bound to be affected if, day after day, you say the opposite of what you feel, if you growl before what you like and rejoice at what brings you nothing but misfortune.

Our nervous system isn't just a fiction; it is part of our physical body, and our soul exists in space and is inside us like the teeth in our mouth. It can't be forever violated with impunity."

—FROM *Doctor Zhivago* BY BORIS PASTERNAK

THE THIRD WAY

WE START BY discussing how combining an understanding of both soma (body) and psyche (mind) can add in a special way to what can be done to help in the recovery from coronary heart disease.

DR DORIAN: Most cardiologists are trained in a scientific model that insists that only what can be accurately measured is important. Measuring psychological well-being is undeniably difficult and, in many respects, imprecise. Together with collaborators, I have become interested in measuring these complex and hard-to-define qualities, such as well-being, and their impact on heart disease. Through my research, I have become convinced that psychological and social aspects of patients' illnesses will influence *not only* how they will feel, but also how they will *be*—in other words, their likelihood of developing further heart attacks or even of dying prematurely. Most importantly, I feel that these aspects can be measured, and that we can use the same scientific tools with which we evaluate, for example, new operations or drugs to evaluate the importance of mood states, attitudes and behaviors on heart disease outcomes. It is in this spirit of using the tools and methods of a scientist, to explore the complex and often murky world of the psyche, that I am collaborating in writing this book.

DR BAKER: But, there is another side to this story. This is not so much the scientific one, but the obvious one; that is, that everybody who has had heart disease, and especially those who have had to deal with the impact of a cardiac event like heart attack, is emotionally affected by it. This cannot be avoided. We are all aware of this, but it is interesting that only recently, with the new findings of research studies that negative emotions can affect cardiac outcome, have cardiologists changed their thinking. On a practical level, though, patients and their families do not have to be convinced that there is an emotional side to this. They know it already.

Dr Dorian: I think this is very clear, even as it was to our grandmothers; however, as a scientist, I am uncomfortable in taking for granted conventional wisdom, even though it seems very sensible and likely to be correct, unless I am able to see some scientific proof of the truth of it. There are, unfortunately, many examples in medicine and other sciences, where concepts, and even treatments, that appear to be correct or effective turn out to be incorrect, and sometimes dangerous. A well-known example comes from the middle of this century, when premature babies were given high-dose oxygen, which turned out to harm rather than help them, causing serious eye problems, completely going against intuition and previous scientific assumption. This is one of many instances where the scientific approach is invaluable in sorting out what is *felt* to be true and that which is, in reality, true.

Dr Baker: We are both committed to this scientific approach, but we must recognize the problem in dealing with matters of the mind. This is the quantifiability question, or "difficulty in measuring" the concepts we are talking about. It is one thing to define an emotional state at a particular time, which we are well able to do in research, but when we are describing, in a broad but meaningful way, the emotional response over time that occurs in the recovery process, it doesn't fit well with research methodology. However, we know enough about the response of patients and their families to convert some of the themes of subjectivity into objective statements. That means we are able to label what people go through, and this, we have found in clinical practice, helps people on the road to recovery.

The field that we are discussing here, involving heart and mind interactions and the close collaboration of cardiac and psychiatric specialties, is relatively new. This book represents an attempt to unify specialties that often operate in isolation. An extra dimension is added, that we feel can help those recovering from a cardiac event.

DR DORIAN: Cardiologists have for many years been primarily interested in the unambiguous "quantity" rather than "quality" of life. What we are trying to suggest is that there is, indeed, a "third way"—namely, taking the best from your understanding of the psychology of the recovery from heart attacks and other heart events, and my cardiologist's understanding of the biology of heart disease and the effect of various drugs and surgical therapies, and by referring to an increasingly sophisticated understanding of the way that the mind and the heart interact. Dr Antonio Damasio, in his intriguing book *Descartes' Error*, explains that not only does the mind control the heart—much as a software controls the computer's output—but that the body itself influences the mind, and that the sensations from the body determine how the mind will react. The research we have collaborated on and other research in this area is beginning to help us unravel precisely what attitudes and behaviors are related to worse cardiac outcome, as much as we have long known that cardiac illness can cause anxiety and depression, difficulty with coping, and so on. A good example is the finding that clinically depressed patients appear to be more vulnerable to death from heart disease and serious heart rhythm disturbances than those not depressed, even with equivalent seriousness of heart disease.

I think you are right in implying that the heart and the mind are constantly performing an intricate and elegant dance, each in turn leading the other, and embracing or more distant, depending on the current rhythm of the body music.

Dr Baker: Well this is music to my ears! I believe we can see this harmony in some of our clinical and research experiences. Two examples are medication compliance and the direct effect of emotion on our patients who have electrical disturbances of the heart.

Dr Dorian: We have shown recently that not only do patients who take their medication as prescribed have a better outcome than those who take only some of their pills, but that this is true even if the patients are administered a placebo (an inactive substance). This tells us that, independent of the treatment itself, being *adherent to treatment* is beneficial. In other words, some psychological or behavioral aspect of being interested in one's own health and actively anticipating in one's treatment protects from heart attack recurrence, and even death, even if that "treatment" is not supposed to be effective! Of course, if the drug treatment *is* effective, which is usually the case, there is that much *more* protection, doubling the reasons to take the medications as prescribed.

Many of our patients with implanted devices to treat serious heart rhythm disorders have their disturbances at times of anxiety or stress. Treating only the consequences of these rhythms may be like adding a fresh coat of paint to an old and crumbling house: it disguises, but does not solve, the underlying problem. Understanding *all* of the causes, including the physical and the psychological, will certainly help our patients to lead happier and healthier lives.

It is perhaps time for us to come full circle in our understanding of how the body and the mind are linked in their response to disease. In spite of initial skepticism some years ago about the influence of one's attitudes and thoughts on one's health, the tools of modern cardiology are now being used to begin to prove what many have suspected: that one's moods, beliefs and attitudes not only help deal with heart disease once it occurs, but also help prevent new complications or recurrences.

DR BAKER: You have strongly emphasized the interactional nature of physical and mental well-being. I will go back to the obvious observation that having heart disease affects one's well-being and that we are now able to describe a sequence that occurs. This sequence is made up of time-dependent phases with which patients can identify. During these phases, certain experiences commonly occur; for example, during recuperation, the body heals. At first, however, an opposite thing is happening in the mind, which starts to *react.* Certain emotional experiences commonly occur, such as depression, which can be a normal response to a cardiac event, but in this case, we have to distinguish between what is "normal" and the severity and persistence that is the hallmark of clinical depression, which does require treatment. In Part One of this book we showed how physical and mental well-being interact, and we tried to communicate to the reader a fusion of cardiac and emotional aspects.

DR DORIAN: This is not a simple "how to" guide. We have tried to explore the terrain between heart and mind, cardiology and psychiatry, in what we hope is an original way.

THEMES OF HEALING

The bumps in the road are not bumps. They are the road.

—Dr Michel Mirowski

In the next "Heart to Mind" dialogue, we examine the different sides of the healing process after a cardiac event, most evident during recuperation. The cardiologist will be seeing the medical component highlighted; whereas the psychiatrist—even one who specializes in dealing with cardiac patients—will still be viewing the other side of the coin. We must remember, though, it's still the same coin! Even though we are specialists, we need to keep in mind we are still treating the same person, and if we can talk to each other as specialists, then we can exchange information, improve communication and, most importantly, treat the whole person.

Dr Baker: "Recuperation" is a big word with a lot of meanings. From the medical standpoint, how do you see it?

Dr Dorian: Literally speaking, Brian, the meaning of "recuperation" is "healing"—in other words, the restoration of the body to its former state of health. After a heart attack, permanent damage actually does occur. Strictly speaking, therefore, a heart can never recover to "completely" normal, or to its previous state. However, there is definitely a process of healing going on after a heart attack, when the heart muscle cells that have died form into a scar. Fortunately, patients can lead reasonably normal and productive lives even when a considerable portion of the heart muscle is scarred. By and large, recuperation consists of initial rest for a few days, followed by a gradual and measured increase in physical and social activities toward normal. This process is a prelude to rehabilitation, whereby many patients can grow even fitter and stronger, physically and psychologically, than they were before their cardiac event.

The process of healing is importantly influenced by medications that are now available to cardiologists, and which can diminish the long-term serious consequences of a heart attack. These medications, such as ACE inhibitors, beta blockers, and ASA, can reduce the severity of heart muscle weakness or enlargement, and the likelihood of short-term complications. It is therefore extraordinarily important for patients to carefully follow their cardiologist's instructions in this early phase.

DR BAKER: I understand that there are many different possible outcomes in this phase. Can you outline what the possibilities are?

DR DORIAN: The traditional concept of having a heart attack, recovery in hospital and at home, and then getting back to one's previous life actually occurs in a minority of patients. These days, especially in the United States (and, to a smaller extent, Canada), many patients undergo intensive investigations immediately after a heart attack or an episode of unstable angina, including *coronary angiography.* Many patients then go on to having *angioplasty* or *coronary bypass surgery* in the days to weeks following their initial episode. The first several months following the acute illness is extremely variable in pattern. Some patients will have their angioplasty or bypass surgery during the first hospitalization, and then face a recovery from the initial event as well as the procedure. Others are discharged home but develop complications in the first days to weeks, and require repeat hospitalization or urgent investigation. Still others feel reasonably well, but investigations show that their long-term outcome can be made more favorable by interventions.

For some patients, therefore, the need for surgery or intensive testing comes as a surprise, which further complicates the process of recovery. For others, a recurrence of symptoms shortly after hospital discharge, or even while in hospital, causes the initial anxiety of the event, which may have decreased, to reemerge, and can lead to a subtle desperation in some. How do you think this "roller coaster" affects patients psychologically?

DR BAKER: The effect on their emotions is prominent. Recuperation is a strange and vulnerable time because patients are going through the various physical responses to the event but at the same time, after the suppression of emotions during the shock phase, a psychological "release" is occurring; that is, they are starting to react emotionally to the event, and this includes experiencing normal fear, anger, low mood and sadness, which can go on for some time. But what can definitely complicate the situation, as we see in the case of Mary, is when patients think they are well and are reminded of their medical state by a recurrence of chest pain or news of an abnormal test result. Maybe this is the time to look at the intersection of heart and mind. There are two situations that I have found to have been neglected by most clinicians. These are the interaction of, first, anxiety and physical symptoms, and second, depression and fatigue.

Once the doctor has given reassurance, the patient feels relieved. However, many patients start to have their symptoms again, such as chest pain, palpitations or shortness of breath. At this point, they have problems interpreting what this means. The obvious concern is that they are again experiencing a threat, and the response is one of anxiety. The big conundrum is that anxiety itself can produce the same symptoms as these cardiac complaints! The question of whether a patient is anxious or physically symptomatic is a difficult one. I have the advantage of having all my patients "cleared" from a cardiac perspective, but it remains a considerable challenge to sort out, as patients can still get ill, even after medical reassurance has been given. Patients need to recognize their symptoms and watch for any change in them; but, in particular, they need to recognize what anxiety is for them and know that, once they have learned to calm down—even with the help of a tranquilizer on rare occasions if necessary—they can then determine to what extent their symptoms were anxiety-related. Certainly it never pays to be anxious or to overreact; not that people want to be this way, but they need to be reminded that it can only aggravate the situation. Have you come across this problem in your clinical practice?

Dr Dorian: Absolutely. Often it is very difficult to distinguish the psychological component from the physical component of symptoms. I am personally convinced that almost all physical symptoms are the result of some abnormal physical sensation that patients are actually feeling. Mild sensations may be amplified and interpreted by the emotional brain to be very unpleasant, and even devastating. I call this concept, borrowing from research on pain thresholds, "somatic amplification." In some senses, it may be impossible to distinguish in individual patients what portion of a symptom is anxiety-related and what portion is "heart-related." What we can do reliably, however, is measure accurately what the cardiac prognosis is in a given individual. We can, for example, establish that a given person has only a small amount of heart muscle "at risk," and therefore even if he or she keeps having chest pain, the risk of another major heart attack is small.

Or, in another example, a patient may have some heart damage but not too much. Shortness of breath or fatigue in these individuals is likely in only a small measure caused by their heart muscle weakness, and, to a larger degree, caused by the emotional consequences of their heart disease.

Our research has shown that subjective fatigue and shortness of breath is an extremely important determinant of the likelihood of dying after a heart attack. Somewhat surprisingly, however, the extent of shortness of breath and fatigue is not clearly related to the severity of heart scarring or the size of the heart attack, implying that the way in which the brain interprets signals from the body has an important effect on how patients will do in the future. It has been known for a long time that the extent of heart damage is itself not closely related to the ability to perform physical activities, further underlying the concept that it's not how bad your heart is, but what you can do with it, that is important.

Can you speculate on what it is that makes subjective fatigue so potentially harmful?

DR BAKER: The question of fatigue and depression is one that is confronting clinicians and researchers from various specialties at this very moment. Many things contribute toward fatigue. Depression is not the whole story, but a significant one, that at least has the benefit of being very responsive to treatment. In the case of Joe, we can see how long it took for his fatigue to be recognized as a symptom of clinical depression, which, if left untreated, has potentially serious consequences, including a poorer cardiac outcome. Luckily, in Joe's case, he had a condition that was finally recognized and was completely treatable.

Perception varies from one individual to the next. When a symptom is perceived, one can distinguish between two types of interpretation of that symptom. One is called "denotation," which is the direct meaning of the symptom, and the other is "connotation," which is the particular association the individual has for it. It is that second one that can give rise to all types of problems, because the association can be much exaggerated. We can see that in the case of Kevin, who represents a sensitive individual. With sensitivity comes reactivity; if you are too sensitive, you can overreact, which, in turn, can complicate your original problem.

Dr Dorian: The good news in all of this is that many patients, even with relatively severe heart damage, *can lead active, productive lives*, despite the severity of their underlying heart scarring. I have many patients whose heart, on paper, looks very poor indeed, but actually are leading satisfying lives of high quality, with only modest limitations. There is no question that anxiety or worry about one's condition tends to be counterproductive. Bobby McFerrin, in his song "Don't Worry, Be Happy," expressed this rather nicely in the line: "In every life there is some trouble; if you worry, you'll make it double." I firmly believe that when patients become anxious, their body sends signals to their brain that the brain has a hard time distinguishing from signals coming from the heart that actually indicate malfunction. It is therefore important and useful for patients to learn to distinguish bodily sensations that are related to their heart from general bodily feelings, which can be done with practice, and education from their doctors and caregivers. Sensations that are not related to the heart can give rise to considerable distress. Such distress may prevent them from engaging in the very heart-healthy habits that can lead to their effective recovery.

Dr Baker: One of the big problems with trying to simplify the journey of recovery is cutting it up into segments. I am sure that many will realize that the process of recuperation will not end at one point and rehabilitation start without any trace of what preceded it. What is your view about how recuperation reaches its conclusion?

Dr Dorian: I agree with you that it is not a seamless transition from one phase to another. Many patients recuperate, only to be "set back" by new events. Furthermore, recuperation continues for quite some time, even after rehabilitation has begun. These days, rehabilitation begins, in a sense, within hours to days after the acute event, as patients are rapidly discharged from hospitals and receive instructions about diet, smoking cessation, exercise programs and the like. It is therefore clear that the processes of recuperation and rehabilitation are sometimes simultaneous, and sometimes one goes back and forth between these phases.

Generally speaking, most patients will undergo all of the tests and procedures that they are likely to have within a few months of an event like a heart attack or unstable angina. By approximately three to six months, the "smoke" will largely have cleared, and they are not very likely to require rehospitalization. At this stage, they will need to perform the important preparation for their long-term rehabilitation. It is very important to note that the process of entering and continuing rehabilitation should not be a passive one, in other words, something that is "done to" the patient. In order to get successful benefit from rehabilitation, patients need to be actively engaged in the program, need to understand why the various activities that are required are being suggested, and, most importantly, need to be fully convinced that they both want and need rehabilitation.

Dr Baker: We know that the end of recuperation is in sight *when a balance has been achieved.* By this I mean that there is a subsidence of emotional reaction, that patients start to feel more confident within themselves and this usually goes along with a subsidence, or at least stabilization, of their physical symptoms. At the same time one notices a balance occurring within their family or social system as well. This is a preparatory stage to that of rehabilitation.

DR DORIAN: Allow me to say something more about equilibrium. Sometime after the heart attack, or a serious heart event such as unstable angina, many patients have a phase of bewilderment and despair since they perceive themselves to be on a continuous downhill course. However, most patients do achieve some equilibrium after the event. This new equilibrium may seem initially to be at a lower physical level than before the event, but importantly their ability to engage in their usual physical and social activities is generally not impaired. In other words, the new equilibrium does not mean that you can no longer do the things that you once loved or liked to do (except of course smoking cigarettes, or eating large amounts of saturated fats!); for many individuals, in fact, recovery and rehabilitation can actually result in a state of well-being that is an improvement over what it was at the time of the original event.

READY FOR REHABILITATION

Men must endure
Their going hence, even as their coming hither
Ripeness is all

—King Lear

The final "Heart to Mind" is about the important phase of rehabilitation. We know that it can be a positive, upbeat phase; but in the real world we all have our aches and pains, our imperfections and flaws. It is hard for us to know when we can move on. So, we have found that a key question during rehabilitation is: When are we ready? This discussion takes advantage of our separate specialties to try to find out more about readiness for rehabilitation.

Dr Baker: Let's start by raising the controversial point that, in fact, rehabilitation commenced just after the cardiac event occurred. If this is so, what distinguishes the rehabilitation phase as we discuss it in this book?

Dr Dorian: Most laypersons, and even cardiologists, think of rehabilitation as simply some sort of structured exercise program, visits with dietitians, exhortations to stop smoking, and so on; these aspects are, of course, very important. However, I think the most important part of rehabilitation is in fact in your realm—psychosocial recovery. In my experience, and our research would tend to support this, rehabilitation only really works if patients are sufficiently psychologically and emotionally prepared to take charge of their own illness, so to speak, as this allows them to follow the program appropriately.

To emphasize the importance of active participation in your own treatment, research results show that patients who, as part of a research study, are assigned to take a placebo and do not take their placebo medications in the proper fashion have a much higher chance of dying than those who do take their placebo. This is clearly not due to a matter of protection supplied by the medication; rather, it speaks to the protection afforded by taking one's medical care seriously. Whatever it is that causes people not to take their pills, including forgetfulness, neglect, loss of concentration and lack of interest in their own health, it is certainly associated with poor outcomes.

Rehabilitation is therefore not simply something that is done to patients, as an organized program months after the heart attack. It begins as soon as you are discharged from the hospital, and have to think about changing your heart habits, perhaps rearranging your schedule to incorporate regular physical activity, changes in your diet and other lifestyle changes.

In this book, we view rehabilitation as that phase that occurs once patients have decided for themselves that they wish to embark on this positive and even liberating journey, which will lead not only to making the most of what they have, but also to improving the quality of their own lives.

DR BAKER: I am interested to hear a cardiologist speak like this. I was always somewhat hesitant in exhorting patients to take the healthy "fork in the road," to push aside ongoing symptoms they may have, and to avoid the sick role. I wondered how much of this was actually in the person's control. One is not always sure how to gauge the empowerment people can actually feel, but, once the empowerment is there, there is a magical quality to this sense of mastery that allows patients to move on with their rehabilitation.

DR DORIAN: How do patients know when they are *emotionally ready for the programs*? For example, many patients are depressed early after heart attacks. How do we integrate our knowledge about depression to recommending programs, which they may not be ready to accept?

DR BAKER: Even if depression is recognized (which it often is not), and treatment commenced, it will take some weeks before the patient starts to feel consistently better. I am referring here to clinical depression; when it is treated, mood and concentration are improved, and motivation can be sustained. Such patients are eligible for the rehab programs. One of the big problems are those patients who suffer from ongoing low mood, which is regarded as "normal" by themselves and others, as they have tended to be somewhat unhappy or "negative" people for a number of years. They tend to go untreated and are probably less likely to participate in rehabilitation programs than their counterparts. A third but overlapping group are those who suffer from fatigue of uncertain origin. Many of these patients may be depressed and are obviously less motivated to participate actively in their rehabilitation than the usual patient.

This book should help people to identify what they are going through on the journey from event to recovery. Once one's emotional response is recognized as being normal under the circumstances, one will not overreact, and when the emotions subside, this is usually the time for the person to "pick up the reins" and take charge of things again. The adage that a journey is a series of single steps is important to remember; when we can demonstrate that we are able to do something, we are more likely to do it again. So, confidence and effectiveness are built on the road to recovery.

DR DORIAN: Brian, it is clear to me, and I think to you, where we would like our patients to "end up" emotionally, socially and physically on this positive journey toward recovery and reintegration. Shouldn't our readers be also concerned about how they *actually get there*? We have described in some detail a state of "being" in which there is a sense of balance, mastery and understanding of one's illness. However, merely knowing the goal may not be enough to allow our patients to get to this state of equilibrium.

DR BAKER: I am pleased that you raised this point, as I am really a pragmatic psychiatrist at heart! I think that other books possibly err on the side of being too much framework and too little soul, but I don't want to get into the problem of the reverse situation. There is the danger of too much exhortation and too little substance. While it is important to give encouragement, and even inspiration, this cannot be done in a vacuum; rather, it must be formulated in the context of what the patient actually goes through after a cardiac event and must be tailored to each individual's particular situation.

From the medical standpoint, how do we judge *readiness for structured activity*, which is the hallmark of rehabilitation?

DR DORIAN: Cardiologists, in general, perform exercise testing to estimate how much "physical work" a patient can safely perform. Fortunately, perhaps surprisingly, almost all patients can safely perform at an intensity that allows them to do all of the activities of daily living. This includes walking about the house, going out to visit friends or to the movies or to the theater, cooking, light housecleaning, going for walks, and even sexual activity. For many patients whose jobs are sedentary, there is no physical reason for them not to return to work. The considerations in respect to activities of daily living are not exclusively "physical." Cardiologists are therefore not as well equipped as we would like to be to know when a patient is ready to go back to work and to resume social, sexual and other activities, except that, in most cases, they can certify that these activities are likely to be safe. Importantly, just because the patients are not in danger doesn't mean that they can resume or begin these activities without effort. Much of this effort is energy wasted in worry. This is not to say worry is abnormal or unusual, but that worry is not *useful* in getting you back to your normal life.

DR BAKER: I often see patients who feel they cannot work, and yet their counterparts with the same degree of cardiac problems are reporting no problems in working. This becomes difficult to evaluate, as we have to go by what the patient tells us. You are touching on a sensitive area in the evaluation of the cardiac patient after a cardiac event, because there are so many reasons why patients do not get motivated to attend their program and return to work. There may be underlying anxiety, fear of performance, depression or whatever. For most cases, it seems clear that patients are not "putting it on." Many are unwilling to return to work for a combination of reasons. One realistic possibility is that the only earnings they are receiving are disability payments, which will cease once they attempt to return to work. We need to be more vigilant about phasing people back into structured activity, to allow them the possibility of a graded return, and protection should they not be able to perform at work.

CHAPTER 12

Six Journeys

Everybody's different. In "The Guide," we took you through what is common for many, if not most, in their journeys of recovery after a cardiac event. However, there are certain types of individuals who show certain types of responses, and one way to reveal what happens with them is to learn about their particular stories. You have been introduced to our "Select Six" in Part One. Here, we give you the opportunity to find out more about their journeys. Through a series of "snapshots" taken during the phases in their journeys, we pick up their stories, starting with the phase (chapter) where you were introduced to each of them—except for our final patient, Kevin. We take you through all the phases of Kevin's journey leading up to his recovery (see Chapter 7).

To obtain a complete picture for each patient, you should review the appropriate sections in Part One before reading this chapter.

TONY: "WHAT—ME WORRY?"

(See also Chapter 2)

Event: What happened to Tony?

Tony was having a drink after dinner when he began to feel unwell—sweaty, short of breath, with an ache between his shoulder blades. His wife quickly noticed that he looked ill and insisted on taking him to the hospital. Through all this, Tony was somewhat oblivious. He thought: "I'll be fine. It's just minor indigestion." He could see that his wife was very concerned.

Although it was quickly established that Tony had had a heart attack, he wasn't really sure what this meant. Within a couple of days, his doctor reassured them that he was now in the clear and he was ready to be discharged home from the hospital. He expected to get back to normal life right away.

There are different forms of the shock response and Tony typifies one end of the spectrum (Kevin, the other). He doesn't know what has hit him. He is also greatly helped by a supportive spouse, who, in a sense, does the worrying *for* him. The role of the significant others is very important during the event, and they either can be a great help or can potentially aggravate the situation. Tony's wife is appropriately concerned, though Tony does rely on her a lot, maybe too much for his own good.

Aftermath: Where is Tony?

Tony and his wife attended the information sessions at the hospital. Before he knew it, he was back home. He wasn't sure what to do with himself. He noticed the cigarette pack in his drawer, but for the moment, he shut it out of his mind. Besides, his wife kept a watchful eye over him. If he started to eat snack foods, she would admonish him with a look or comment. That was all that was needed, and he desisted. He did *feel at loose ends.* He *wasn't too worried, so what was* she *so upset about?*

Tony continues in his fairly oblivious way, but at this point does feel disoriented, being in unfamiliar territory with no particular focus.

There is a tendency to revert to old patterns, even though, of all the phases subsequent to the event, the aftermath is the one where motivation is usually very high. Motivation is propelled by the recent event, like a heart attack, and is heightened during this brief, vulnerable period. Incidentally, smokers who are strongly addicted may still have a tough time here, as one of the cues to smoke is a state of "edge" or slight nervousness, something we can expect even Tony to be feeling. Most, though, will be on their best behavior, especially with their spouses nearby!

All of our "Select Six" are subject to the vigilant or protective response that we have described. However, there are variations that do make a difference. Tony's wife seems watchful and supportive in a relatively uncomplicated way, even though Tony is not too interested in being fussed over. This is fine for this brief stage, but if it continues in this way he may be less independent or more resentful than we would like him to be at the end of the journey.

Recuperation: What is Tony going through?

Tony couldn't help being wary these days, what with his wife and the doctor giving all this advice! But he just wanted to get back to his life. He had found that he felt better when preoccupied in his tool shed or when he watched the sports channel. He thought: If I get stronger, I can get back to work.

Even Tony goes through some form of fear, which can be normal at this time. In Tony's case, he is keen to find a diversion as he is uncomfortable facing his situation and confronting his feelings, which are well hidden from view. Work can provide a focus, but if these underlying feelings persist, they need to be dealt with; otherwise, Tony will likely have difficulties.

In those early weeks after his heart attack, Tony momentarily thought that he wouldn't get well again. He also briefly doubted he could return to his job in the parts department, especially when he wasn't feeling well, as he was when he was started on medication that didn't agree with him. But before long he would distract himself, or his wife would offer a supportive comment. It also bothered him when his sexual performance was not what it used to be, but his family doctor had reassured him this was normal and would improve with time.

It is part of the normal response after a cardiac event to feel low, down or blue. This seems directly related to not being "yourself," particularly in terms of the ability to resume normal activities. As time goes on, many of these inabilities fade as you see that in fact you *can do* what you thought you could not in those early days of recuperation. It is extremely helpful to have supportive people around, and Tony is fortunate to have such a person in his wife. The family physician can also be helpful in giving reassurance. Should the low mood persist, this must be evaluated to rule out clinical depression or persistent low mood (see Chapters 5 and 10).

Rehabilitation: What is Tony doing?

As time went on, Tony became more and more involved in his work and his previous interests: watching the sports channel, drinking beer and smoking cigarettes. He would do some fixing in the garage or the basement, but the only real exercise he got was walking their rather lethargic dog around the block. It was at those times that chest pain would emerge and Tony would slow down to allow it to subside. He had dropped out of the rehab program, but he felt reasonably well, he thought. He could see that his wife was unhappy with him, but she knew not to nag him about it.

Another form of slippage is not complying with your treatment recommendations. This can occur almost without being noticed, as is the case with Tony, although certainly not with his wife, who has, however, learned that she will not get anywhere by constantly reminding him. Tony is slowly starting to "stack the odds" against a good recovery and increasing the chances of a recurrent cardiac event, which could be a threat to him.

Recovery: Has Tony recovered?

Tony attended his follow-up with the cardiologist, and everything seemed stable. He nodded affirmatively when asked if he would try harder to stick to the exercise and dietary guidelines, from which he knew he had strayed completely. He promised to do his best to stop smoking. Once he left the office, he gave a sigh and then thought of other things. His wife, who had waited in the car, wondered what Tony had told the doctor. She knew not to nag him, but he simply was ignoring the fact of being a heart patient. In one sense it was admirable: he just did what he liked. Unfortunately, what he liked was not good for him.

We are now very familiar with Tony's problem and we know that it is an understatement to say that maintenance is "a challenge" in his case. But Tony's story makes the point strongly: we will easily lapse into bad habits unless we develop good ones to replace them! Tony may be blissfully unaware of what he is ignoring, but his wife is not. However, she has discovered that he will retreat further if she keeps reminding him of what he should and should not do. Awareness and motivation must come from within, but this does not mean that we cannot help someone to become aware and motivated. In this book, we have attempted to develop this by explaining what the underlying process is, from event to recovery. The media and the medical profession have become much more vocal in declaring the message about heart health. Hopefully this will get through to the Tonys of the world.

ANNA: "REPEATED EPISODES"

(See Chapter 3.)

Aftermath: Where is Anna?

This was the third time Anna was home from the hospital. Now, *she had been told, she would be fine. Being a person who secretly mistrusted others, it was hard for her to believe that. After all her experiences over the past months, she knew that one is expected to feel a little strange and vulnerable at times like this and that, in spite of her doubting nature, the feeling would probably pass.*

Anna's husband, who didn't usually pay her much attention, was around much more and seemed more interested in her well-being. Now that *she welcomed.*

The aftermath phase is a trying time that will pass, but seems endless. Anna, who has been through two previous cardiac events, is beset by strange or discordant feelings. Patients are subject to the vigilant or protective response that is so characteristic for this phase. In the case of Anna, the marriage is being affected by the course of her heart disease. After three hospitalizations, there seems to be a "drawing in" of her husband back into his wife's life. Anna's story has become complicated by the repeated cardiac episodes, and it is during the aftermath that the uncertainty looms. It is very reassuring for Anna, whose mistrust of the world has not been helped by recurrent heart problems, to have a close person provide emotional support, and even more so if it could signal that the marriage is coming together again.

Recuperation: What is Anna going through?

Anna tried to settle herself down. She didn't have pain anymore, but sometimes after brooding on what had happened she noticed some tightness in her chest. The doctor had said she was medically stable. But how could she know what would happen? She had already had one heart attack, and then two angioplasty procedures. The last time she checked with the doctor, she was told that anxiety could be contributing to her symptoms. How was she to know what was nerves and what was real?

Almost everyone can identify with Anna as she wonders about her chest pain. In the healing process, the body goes through its adjustments. There often are *some* symptoms, be they chest pain, fatigue, shortness of breath or palpitations. The question then becomes: What do they *mean*? Anna will know that it is not easy for "the patient" to self-diagnose. The choices are varied, and so are the implications. On the one hand, the symptoms may have little consequence: they may mean nothing (say, a muscular pain), or they may mean something (say, surgery effect) but nothing needs to be done. On the other hand, the symptoms could mean that medical attention is needed—perhaps immediately. Even qualified cardiologists do not always know what to do. The severity of pain is not necessarily related to the severity of the situation; with the advice of their doctors, patients need to learn how to interpret the symptoms *particular* to them.

To top things off, anxiety itself can give rise to the *same* symptoms that we see after a cardiac event—chest pain, shortness of breath, lack of concentration, and a cold, clammy feeling. As anxiety can occur in response to a threat, a perceived threat in the form of physical symptoms will trigger anxiety, setting in motion a "vicious circle." We need to avoid this potential spiral by recognizing and dealing with it when it occurs.

In the weeks after her third hospitalization, Anna went through more emotions than was usual for her. It was true that her physical symptoms had waned, but she still felt insecure. This was mixed with some bitterness about her condition and what would happen to her in the future. Over the years Anna had become quite disgruntled with her lot in life. She had ended up spending most of her time at the dry-cleaning business. She'd always had a tendency to be mistrustful of others: What could you expect? People were always taking advantage. She could give you many examples to prove this. A creeping cynicism that had developed over the years wasn't helped much by what she had gone through these past few months. Two things were buoying her spirits now: as time progressed she did feel stronger; also, her husband seemed genuinely interested in her and—surprise, surprise—was even affectionate toward her.

Here it is revealed that over the years Anna has become disgruntled, mistrustful and cynical about people. If such patients have experienced a cardiac event, and particularly if stabilization of their medical state has for some reason been delayed, as in the case of Anna, bitterness and anger felt inwardly or expressed outwardly can be expected. Once her physical state has become stabilized and rehabilitation commenced, a subsidence of her "edge" can be expected, but, given what we now know, anger and her mistrustful attitudes are liable to continue, and anger management (see Chapter 10) may be a helpful alternative. Anna's negative feelings are somewhat mitigated by an increasing closeness within her marriage.

Rehabilitation: What can Anna do?

Anna was finding out that there was more to herself than she had previously realized. This whole anger thing was a revelation to her. She had just kept her irritations and bitterness to herself, thinking this was just her, *and nothing could be done about it. Over the months she and her husband had been followed up by their family doctor, an experienced therapist who had helped her, and had brought her and her husband together so that they could air their grievances. They had learned not to stop fighting, but rather to fight more effectively! Along the way, Anna had attended an assertiveness course, where she had found out about better ways to express herself and to get what she wanted. She was also not overloading herself at the family business. What with her health not acting up anymore, Anna was going through a real change.*

Anna is becoming more aware of her self, her needs, her emotions, especially anger, her health and her marriage. Quite a task! She is considerably helped by regular follow-ups with her therapist, who is also her family doctor, and the assertiveness course helps her to channel her anger in a way that is constructive. The couples sessions allow an opening up of the communication channels with her husband. However, we cannot expect that these interventions will miraculously solve problems that were years in the making. We can see, though, that here the cardiac event has spurred changes that can have long-lasting positive effects on both Anna and her husband.

Recovery: Is Anna well again?

It dawned on Anna that months had gone by and she had remained relatively well. The three admissions to the hospital had made a mark on her consciousness and she wasn't eager to get on that roller coaster again.

Running a dry-cleaning business was tiring, but the message had gotten through to her brothers. They stipulated that the time at work would be strictly shared, and if they noticed that she looked exhausted again, they were now prepared to take over. They had taken her for granted before, and this included her grumbling. That's just Anna, they thought. But now they noticed that she was more self-assured—as did her husband, who had become so much more involved in the marriage. He watched her more in a caring way, but had learned not to be overprotective of her. He thought to himself that he had also been through a lot, and it was only now, about a year after her first heart attack, that things seemed "normal" again.

Anna is someone who had repeated symptoms of the heart, necessitating hospitalizations. Eventually her health problems subsided, followed by healing and recovery. Anna's loved ones have naturally been affected by this process. At work, her brothers have started to adjust to a new arrangement. Over time, the siblings had begun to take one another for granted, as the grind of long-standing partnership issues got in the way. Now they were adopting a more caring approach toward her.

Anna's husband has been through a transformation himself. He had had to deal with repeated threats to his wife, although it had now been months since there had been any sort of crisis. The marriage was now strengthened. He was determined to ensure that she remain well and that, importantly, they understood each other clearly and were able to articulate any concerns that could develop. Anna's bitterness seemed to have subsided and he was thankful for that. Now they were looking forward to other things. While the old story was not forgotten, Anna and her husband were entering a new chapter of their lives.

ROSE: "WHEN YOU DON'T GET BACK TO NORMAL"

(See Chapter 4.)

Recuperation: What is Rose going through?

It dawned on Rose that this would be a new chapter in her life. She was not as strong as she had been before, though she was told by her doctors that she would improve. But she realized her beloved job was over. She knew she had to retire at some point, in any case, but still it was disappointing. Nevertheless, she wasn't one to dwell on things, and the sadness would waft over her and away from her like a feathery cloud.

Sadness is a normal response after a cardiac event. As we explained in Chapter 5, it is a response to loss, which in most cases turns out to be perceived and not real. The word "grief" can be used, in the sense that something is missed that seems irretrievable. Rose does exemplify this, although we don't know to what extent she will be rehabilitated. While many find that their perception of loss was unfounded, others inevitably do experience some losses. For Rose, there is no doubt that her working days are over. There are other signs that she may well not be "herself" again, and she is correct in assessing this.

Rehabilitation: What did Rose do?

It hadn't been easy. Rose's oldest daughter contemplated the past few months since her mother collapsed in the shopping mall. For the family, the first few weeks had been the most onerous by far, but the subsequent period of recovery had also been a strain. Thankfully, her mother had been making slow but steady progress. It was quite remarkable, if you thought about it. But Rose's daughter had not let on to her mother what the family had quietly gone through. Yes, Rose was admirably independent, almost stubbornly so, but the truth was that she was in large part still quite reliant on her two daughters who lived in town. She had her activities, such as playing cards with her friends, but she didn't really have close friends. During this time, Rose's older daughter had been struggling with her *older daughter, a stubborn teenager—not that unlike her grandmother, come to think of it! Rose's recovery had been slow, but now finally she seemed to be rehabilitated. That was a relief.*

Here we focus on the impact on the family who had quietly accommodated the demands placed on them. Such demands can be burdensome in the first few weeks, particularly in Rose's case, where there is extra concern about whether she will recover at all, or to a state of independent living. Rose's daughters bore their responsibilities in a stoic manner, but we have raised the question (see Chapter 6) about whether the family is supported themselves. Rose's daughters have their own family issues, and they have to contend with these while at the same time keeping an eye on their mother. Should demands be too great, a support group, or even family counseling, can take the pressure off and provide much-needed support to family members.

Recovery: Is Rose well again?

Rose thought about the time since the "shopping-mall incident," as she was prone to call her heart attack and cardiac arrest. So much had changed since then. At first, she had wondered whether she would really emerge from it all, especially in those days when she felt so weak and her daughters were staying with her. After that, it had been a very slow process. She had always prized her independence and was able to keep it, but something her older daughter had recently said reminded Rose that, in fact, she had relied on her family a fair amount. She now appreciated this more than before, because, in truth, she wasn't as independent as she had previously been. Her doctor had put her on a gradual exercise program, and Rose had gained strength over time. She was less physically capable than before, but she had changed her life accordingly. It was a restricted life, but rather good in quality. Although her health was not as good as before the event, it was *stable and she didn't worry much about it. Rose left that to the doctors!*

Rose's acceptance of her current status is a boon to her management. From a health point of view, she is not the person she once was, but she does not dwell on that. Rose is in a state of "adaptive denial" as she takes her medications, does her exercises and generally follows her doctor's instructions. She also has devoted daughters to ensure that she always attends appointments. Rose has slowly come to realize that she is not as independent as she had thought, and that her family had for some time been complicit in masking this. Instead of being upset about it, Rose is thankful. Not all are as accepting as Rose of all the changes that may be required. Once recovered, many will return to a quality of life similar to that before the cardiac event; others will return to a noticeably different status, but nevertheless the quality of life can still be very satisfactory, especially with a positive attitude, as we see with Rose.

MARY: "MS BUSY"

(See Chapter 5.)

Recuperation: What is Mary going through?

Mary was trying to get on with her busy life. For the most part, she could do what she had to do, but tiredness still held her back, and this frustrated her, even getting her down. She had less motivation for work, even for enjoyable activities. Taking any initiative seemed really hard. She couldn't help thinking of her "old self"; she would never have been so incapable before. She had always coped with her heavy load of responsibilities and desires. Mary squeezed a lot into her daily schedule. She had always worked hard; now she had to ensure her children's needs were met, that she found time for her boyfriend, and attend the rehab program too! Mary was finding she just couldn't do everything, and this frustrated and demoralized her.

At times, the distinction between sadness and low mood becomes blurred. Both can be present, as with Mary . Your mood goes down when you have the feeling that the world is "on top" of you, rather than the reverse. You cannot control "it"; it controls you. In the early stages in the recovery from a cardiac event like heart attack, this feeling is common and can be quite normal. Mary has many responsibilities, which she doesn't usually shirk. She thrives on being busy. By this time, though, both her body and mind are on a "go slow," if not on an outright strike. When her one focus in life—her activities—are threatened, it is not surprising that frustration and unhappiness take hold.

Many patients like Mary will go through normal periods of sadness relating to what has happened, and low mood relating to feelings of incapacity; over time, these feelings will subside; flare-ups, though, are to be expected. Depression and fatigue is a pattern that is now being better recognized (see Chapter 5, Chapter 10, and Chapter 11, "Themes of Healing").

Rehabilitation: What did Mary do?

After her setback, Mary took stock of her lifestyle. "Busy as a bee," they used to say about her. She had gotten so used to running on adrenaline; she now realized she was almost addicted to it. Mary had to admit that she had mostly loved it, but that it wasn't doing her much good. She had so many responsibilities—some of them related to her great competence at her job. Since the heart attack, she had started to reevaluate how she would now run her life. Her priorities were changing: she had learned to give more time to her children (when they had time for her!), her boyfriend and number one—herself!

Mary has experienced a setback, but this has forced her to take stock of the way she is conducting her life. Much of this relates to the way she "paces" it. The problem is that she usually thrived on being busy; now her body had given notice that, at least in the recovery process, she should not push herself. (There is not necessarily a link of her lifestyle to heart disease—see Chapter 5). Maybe, she could use this over time to take stock of her life in general. We don't expect her to change completely; also her job depends to a certain extent on her considerable capacities. But now Mary is starting to apportion more time to her loved ones, and ultimately to benefit herself.

Recovery: Is Mary well again?

"I shouldn't be doing this," Mary told herself as she took on another project. The trouble was, she was so good at what she did! On all other levels, the year had ended so amazingly differently from the beginning, when her life was rudely interrupted by her heart attack. The wedding had gone smoothly, and her teenagers were apparently getting along well with her new husband. Everyone seemed to be open about their feelings and opinions.

Mary had made big changes in her daily routines and her life generally. She was dedicated to keeping herself healthy. She enjoyed her exercise, and with the help of her medications and keeping to her low-fat diet, her cholesterol was getting into the normal range. Within herself, her spiritual side had been awakened, and her husband shared this with her. Generally, she felt more centered than before, but her underlying restlessness and desire to keep focused remained. Oh well, she thought, there's another challenge for me!

"When you go away, you always have to take yourself along"—so goes the old adage. Recovery does not occur in a vacuum. We all have our own issues and tendencies. There is nothing abnormal about this. Mary made a good recovery, once she had gotten over her setbacks. As it happened, it was not only her health that was out of balance, but also other aspects of her life. Now, she is more in tune with her children and is dedicated to putting her life back into a state of inner and outer harmony. However, changing character is more easily said than done, and Mary retains the need to keep focused and busy. This is not necessarily bad for her, as long as she does not seriously overload herself. However, she studiously deals with her main risk factors, and she now recognizes that, with a family history, it is important that her children also see and get used to an environment that is conducive to a heart-healthy lifestyle.

Happily, as she enjoys exercise, and her diet as well, this lifestyle is not a problem for her.

JOE: "JOE IS STALLED"

(See Chapter 5, for introduction and comment on depression, and Chapter 6, for forum.)

Joe just couldn't see the bright side. The future seemed bleak; he criticized himself for weakness. Later, during moments of clarity, he realized that this was unfair, but for the most part, he just couldn't help himself. His main problem, though, was that he found it hard to get himself going. This state lasted for weeks. He had little interest and pleasure in things, things he usually loved to do, and his thinking was slow. He was being "carried" at work, but his partners didn't complain about this. Joe, however, was sure that at some point they would just get fed up with him and fire him from the partnership.

Joe's wife received a telephone call from a colleague of Joe's: "I am sure he is depressed. He reminds me so much of my brother who was similar to Joe, and he recovered after treatment. He is not doing work around the office anyway. Please ask him to see his doctor." The penny had dropped! Joe's wife called the family doctor, whom they knew well, and that day he confirmed their suspicions. He asked her to see his colleague, a psychiatrist, who was soon explaining that Joe had a clinical depression, which required and should respond to treatment. This consisted of one of the newer antidepressants as well as ongoing talking treatment and monitoring. A cardiologist was consulted, and Joe was started on an antidepressant, to be evaluated on a weekly basis. He was to call if there were any problems. Side effects were quite possible, especially in the early days, and if they were prominent or persistent, the medication would have to be changed.

Joe felt a sense of relief as he realized that this explained so much of what he had gone through over the weeks since the heart attack. Now he had something else! Still, he was reassured that there was light at the end of the tunnel. Within himself, though, he still felt exactly as before—just as bad—but the knowledge that he had something that he was told should respond to treatment did boost his spirits, even if only superficially.

Joe has developed a clinical depression that has eventually been recognized and treated. Joe has started to show a response, but he must wait some weeks before the full effect of the treatment can be felt. He benefits from the talking part of the treatment as well (psychotherapy), and this can be invaluable in the early stages before the medication has "kicked in." His cardiac state was taken into consideration before starting the antidepressant. Joe may have been considered for a particular type of psychotherapy—cognitive therapy—but we have found that this type is more effective in treating the milder forms of clinical depression or persistent low mood (for details, see Chapters 6 and 10).

Recovery: Is Joe well again?

Joe surveyed the past year. Most of the time his heart attack seemed far away; with reminders, it loomed overhead. He had become familiar with his extraneous heartbeats. But he was ready to deal with any eventuality. He felt physically quite strong and was pleased that he still exercised regularly. He took his medications, but at times he would have lapses with his low-fat diet; for the most part, though, he followed the guidelines. Joe was an obedient type, as he had discovered in his therapy sessions. He had fully recovered from his depression. It wasn't easy, but he had started to assert himself at work, and even at home. He was surprised that instead of his relationships being threatened, they seemed to improve, and he felt good about this.

Joe's journey had started off as a rough one. Not only did he have the heart attack, but he had a clinical depression, which was initially undiagnosed, as well. However, he had responded to treatment and had benefited greatly from attending the rehab program. Later, he had coped well when he developed a heart rhythm disturbance.

Joe has learned a lot over the past year. He feels on top of things. He knows all about his condition and feels prepared for eventualities. Along the way, he has learned more about himself, and has started to make attempts to improve how he deals with others in his life, such as his spouse and work colleagues. He feels equipped to handle the future. He is recovered.

KEVIN: "MR REACTIVE"

(See Chapter 7.)

Event: What happened to Kevin?

Kevin was gripped with a type of distant terror as it dawned on him that this was an "emergency." His wife kept crying and holding him. They had always been so close, too close, he had thought at times. What was going on? Maybe he was having a heart attack. His father's heart troubles crossed his mind.

A sense of unreality crept over him as the ambulance rushed him to hospital. Fear broke through as he wondered if he would be okay. Time seemed to flip-flop; at times it sped along, at other times it would be at a standstill. The doctor was explaining that they were checking to see if he had had a heart attack. He felt his wife's grip on his hand. Soon he was being told that an emergency angiogram was required, and then bypass surgery recommended. It was all too fast.

When his wife visited after the surgery, he still couldn't quite believe what had happened to him. It was only on the weekend the family had been vacationing and everything had seemed just fine!

Kevin is at the other end of the spectrum of the shock from where Tony was. He is an emotional type. He experiences alarm and shock, as his wife probably does as well, and this reaction was probably intensified by the suddenness of the surgery he has undergone. Postoperatively, Kevin will clearly not be over the shock of this phase.

The role of the significant others is very important during the event, and they can either be a great help or a great hindrance. In the case of Kevin, he and his spouse are so bonded to each other, so "interdependent," that when significant stress occurs there is the danger that the situation can actually be worsened. A "spiral" can occur, with each partner upsetting the other; on the positive side, Kevin and his wife *are* mutually supportive, and, again, in trying to understand a spouse's actions we must keep in mind that he or she is going on a journey as well at this time.

It is Kevin who will have an intense and persistent response during this brief phase and the next, not-so-brief phase. Too much response, and for too long, needs to be dealt with, but having *some* anxiety may help with adherence to treatment, and this, in itself, may lead to a better outcome.

Aftermath: Where is Kevin?

Kevin felt that he was in the twilight zone—everything had changed so much. It was unreal! He was still in some pain from the operation. He would admit it was not severe; it was more that something had been done *to him, and the sensations were strange. He was also having trouble concentrating. It was hard to look at himself in the mirror, his chest, his legs. His wife wouldn't let him out of her sight. He woke up with her staring at him. At times, she seemed more upset than him.*

These situations are typically seen in the aftermath. This trying time will pass, but that is sometimes hard to believe when you are inside this cauldron of confusion. We note the closeness of Kevin's marriage, with the expected "hypervigilant" response of his wife. While this is quite common, we need to watch the watchfulness, to avoid unhealthy patterns being established. In very close couples, there is a strong emphasis on the "we" of the relationship, rather than the "I" or independent side. Ideally, there should be a good balance between these two aspects of the marriage. For the journey of recovery, we watch for subsidence of the protective response, which should occur fairly soon into the next phase.

Recuperation: What is Kevin going through?

Kevin's mind just wouldn't settle down. He kept going over what happened and couldn't stop himself from thinking what might *have happened. This, again, forced him unwillingly to the next topic—what may* still *happen! Would he have a heart attack? One thought was worse than the next!*

Previously, Kevin had never thought of himself as particularly nervous. A thinker, sensitive to the world—yes!—but now, a few weeks after bypass surgery, he felt like a wreck. His hands felt cold, his stomach was in a knot and his muscles were tensed.

He was thankful for the support of his wife and, frankly, quite envious of her. Now she *had started to calm down!*

Kevin illustrates well what is possibly the commonest emotional reaction after a cardiac event—fear. This is a normal response, but in Kevin's case it will be exaggerated. Interestingly, Kevin had not seen himself as "particularly nervous"; however, we suspect that he had this tendency before; the cardiac event has brought out the emotional reaction that can be expected to be strong during the recuperation phase. Kevin shows well the time component of fear, with the emphasis on being shaken by the past and especially by the possibility of something happening in the future (see Chapter 6).

Happily, Kevin's wife is starting to settle down and this can greatly help Kevin to restabilize. The alternative is for both partners to upset each other, creating a "spiral" and worsening recovery for both spouses, something we naturally want to avoid.

"I'll never be the same again." Kevin's mind wouldn't settle down. He was often worried, and when he was not sadness crept over him. Now he was a heart patient! He felt that he was changed forever. That familiar invulnerable self he had always taken for granted was gone. He missed it! He thought of how he had been and how he was now—he was no longer complete. He felt that his position in the marriage was changing: now he would no longer be the confident partner he had been before.

Kevin is saddened by the loss of his old identity; the fact of his now being a "heart patient" is a real issue that will need to be accepted over time, but much of what saddens Kevin is *perceived* and he should adjust in time. Kevin has a tendency to worry, and this will amplify his concerns.

Six weeks since his surgery, Kevin was still not at peace with himself. "Why me?" he thought. Why not those guys he sees at ball games gob-

bling down cheeseburgers? He knew so many people who had lifestyles much less healthy than his. He conceded that he didn't really watch his diet much, and it was true that his father had had his first heart attack in his forties as well, but Kevin wasn't obviously overweight, if you discounted his potbelly, and he hadn't ever smoked. Kevin didn't dwell on these points. They simply crossed his mind and then, with irritation, he silently muttered to himself: "It just isn't fair!"

Kevin goes through what is a common experience for many after a cardiac event—anger as a reaction. "Why me?" is an existential outcry that is easy to understand: so much of what happens seems so unfair! Often, with probing, one discovers that the patient may indeed have been denying certain risk factors and may not have been for regular checkups, but this still does not detract from the fact that others with similar habits do not suffer a cardiac event, at least not now.

With a sympathetic response of spouse, friend or counselor, patients will find that, as long as there is not a history of ongoing anger, the reactive anger will subside over time.

Rehabilitation: What did Kevin do?

As Kevin walked out of the rehab center, he could virtually feel the weight lifting from his shoulders. It was hard to pinpoint when exactly this had occurred. He had been evaluated with various contraptions, had been found eligible to participate and had been given his own personal program. He had talked to other participants, and then they had all attended the opening lecture. In truth, Kevin's emotional state had started to subside some weeks before, but he hadn't yet found a focus for himself. He now felt that he could come out of this, and he could still make a good life for himself, and for his family.

It is not that unusual to find that someone with Kevin's emotional makeup can do well when his energies are harnessed, as it were, in a rehab program. From the start, you can notice an upbeat, positive attitude as there is the sense that you can *do* something about getting better. As you demonstrate your newfound abilities, mastery and empowerment occur (see Chapter 6). For people like Kevin, it is when things don't go well, and also in the long term, that there is a risk of the emotional reaction returning.

Kevin's journey of recovery is highlighted in Chapter 7. We see that Kevin's confidence is now restored and he feels ready for any eventuality. How he actually copes remains to be seen. What we do know is that although Kevin has had to go through difficult times, as is true for Anna, Joe and Mary, the journey has also provided an opportunity to learn and to grow, so as to meet the challenges of journeys to come.

Recommended Reading

Patients and their families are always asking about suitable reading material to help them in the recovery process after the cardiac event. We have found that there is surprisingly little material that is universally embraced, even though there are many pertinent books available. What follows is a *personal* selection. It is neither definitive nor comprehensive, and is based on our own reading of the material, and especially the effect it has had on cardiac patients and their families—namely, to somehow inspire or teach them something that we hold to be important to the recovery process after a cardiac event.

For a basic explanation of how the heart works and the risk factors for heart disease and what you can do about them, the American Heart Association's *Your Heart: An Owner's Manual* (New York: Pocket, 1996) is useful. Its message is conveyed with much clarity, in handbook style, and the facts are presented in a straightforward way. A similar approach is taken in *The USP Guide to Heart Medications* (New York: Avon, 1996).

Perhaps the most widely read books are by Dean Ornish—including his groundbreaking *Stress, Diet and Your Heart* (New York: Signet, 1994) and the best-selling *Dr. Dean Ornish's Program for Reversing Heart Disease* (New York: Ivy, 1996). Dr Ornish's books emphasize a comprehensive programmatic approach, which includes a strong emphasis on diet and stress management and is based on the author's own research studies. Written with irrepressible enthusiasm, they do not address the process of recovery *per se*.

We certainly recommend both the books mentioned here; however, we are not convinced that patients need to follow such a rigorous program, especially in light of our observation that in general they find it difficult to remain on these types of programs.

For a practical guide to a program with specific application to the patient after a cardiac event, see Dr Terence Kavanagh's *Take Heart!* (Toronto: Key Porter, 1992). Kavanagh emphasizes the exercise component, and patients can easily embrace his pragmatic approach to rehabilitation.

Rhoda Levin's *Heartmates: A Survival Guide for the Cardiac Spouse* (Scarborough, ON: Prentice-Hall, 1987) has gained wide recognition for championing the experience of the much-neglected spouse of the patient who has suffered a cardiac event. Based on her own experience, the book illustrates what the spouse goes through, with vignettes that are easy for spouses to identify with. The Heartmates organization has also been established to deal with spousal concerns.

There are few books that deal with the emotional aspects of recovery after a cardiac event that our patients have embraced. For those who wish to embark on the programmatic side, the only one with potential relevance for the cardiac patient is Redford Williams and Virginia Williams's *Anger Kills*. It is written in a simple style and gives readers a chance to rate their anger and learn to deal with it. The flow chart on how to decide what to do when angry is particularly helpful.

Heart-healthy cookbooks have contributed much to the rehabilitation and prevention of CAD, and the cookbooks by Anne Lindsay—*Lighthearted Everyday Cooking* (Toronto: Macmillan, 1991), *New Light Cooking* (Toronto: Ballantine, 1998)—and Bonnie Stern—*Simply Heartsmart Cooking* (Toronto: Random House Canada, 1994), *More Heartsmart Cooking* (Toronto: Random House

Canada, 1997)—have been extremely popular in Canada. The menus are presented in a very engaging way and, importantly, are actually used and greatly enjoyed by readers.

The Healing Heart (New York: Norton, 1983) is an eloquently written personal account of his heart disease by the writer Norman Cousins.

The important issue of "Why me?" after a life-threatening event is cogently dealt with in the justifiably popular *Why Bad Things Happen to Good People* (New York: Schocken, 1981) by Harold Kushner. This is one of the few books that actually inspire and help people in a circumscribed but vital way.

For a basic "in your face" book on assertiveness, *When I Say No I Feel Guilty* by Manuel J. Smith (New York: Bantam, 1985) continues to provoke; it gets across the point that you must stick up for your rights like few other books do.

The Road Less Traveled by M. Scott Peck (New York: Simon & Schuster, 1978) has become legendary in our time. It conveys the basic truth that stress is inevitable and that life is hard in a unique way. There is a depth to the writing that vast numbers of readers find persuasive.

Cognitive therapy has now become well established and is used for a number of emotional problems, especially depression. Even though the material is by nature dense, David Burns's first book, *Feeling Good: The New Mood Therapy* (New York: Signet, 1980), remains popular with readers.

Harriet Lerner's *The Dance of Anger: A Woman's Guide to Changing the Patterns of Intimate Relationships* (New York: Harper & Row, 1986) is extremely effective in describing the common pattern of "pursuer–distancer" in relationships between couples, where one partner is seen as too emotionally demanding by the other, resulting in a vicious circle.

For spiritual guidance, we recommend you refer to whatever works for you and articulates the framework of your spiritual beliefs, giving you spiritual solace and inspiration.

An article by I. Wiklund, H. Sanne, A. Vedin and C. Wilhelmsson titled "Coping with Myocardial Infarction: A Model with Clinical Applications. A Literature Review" in *International Rehabilitation Medicine* 7/4 (1985): 167–75, summarizes a number of concepts related to the emotional impact of heart attack. Wiklund has published extensively on quality of life and medical conditions.

Descartes' Error: Emotion, Reason, and the Human Brain by Antonio R. Damasio (New York: Putnam, 1994) is a lucid, scientifically oriented approach to the links between emotions, feelings, and brain function.

A summary of recent findings on the heart–brain link can be found in *Heart and Mind* by Robert Allen and Stephen Scheidt (Washington, DC: American Psychological Association, 1996).

Glossary

In "The Guide" and "Directions," we repeatedly use a series of words that, in the end, make up the "language" of our message to you, to help you on the journey from cardiac event to recovery. This glossary is a collection of the key words that make up our message to you. In the brief explanation we provide, we try to be as non-technical as we can, but we do expect you to wince on occasion. Never mind, once a word or phrase is imprinted in your brain, it should be there for good!

accommodating: The tendency to yield to others, to allow others to get their way with you, even if you would prefer it the other way around! See also *submissive*.

acetylsalicylic acid (ASA): Well known as aspirin, this commonly used painkiller prevents blood platelets from sticking together and thus delays or prevents clotting of the blood. It is very useful in preventing heart attacks and treating *unstable angina*.

aftermath: The second of the five phases of the journey of recovery. It is a relatively short period of time, often only a few days, and usually corresponds with the patient's return home after a cardiac event, like a heart attack. Family members can show a characteristic protective response toward the patient, which can become exaggerated and cause problems for patient and family. See also *hypervigilance*; *phases*.

aggression: The outward expression of or tendency to show anger. More pointed ways of demonstrating this anger include attacks, hostility or being destructive. See also *anger*; *hostility*.

anger: The feeling that will normally occur if we are threatened, frustrated or disappointed, and if we are in the process of reacting to an event that may have occurred, such as a cardiac event. Anger can therefore be a reaction (see Kevin) or an ongoing tendency (see Anna) that can then be associated with a negative view of the world, including mistrust of people and a general cynical attitude toward the way of the world. Ongoing anger may be a risk factor for CAD. See also *aggression*; *anger management*; *hostility*.

anger management: The systematic attempt to deal with anger. It includes learning to identify what sparks the anger ("the cue") and specifically handling the often strong anger response, usually with suppression (stopping it) or, if the anger is justified, converting it to assertiveness (see below) so as to achieve what you think you deserve. See also *stress management*.

angina: Pain, discomfort or pressure, usually in the chest, back, upper arms or jaw, caused by an insufficient blood supply to the heart muscle. Literally, it means "pain." Sometimes lack of blood supply to the heart is experienced as nausea, dizziness or shortness of breath, which is called "atypical angina."

angiogram: An X-ray test to examine blood vessels, involving the injection of dye into an artery (blood vessel), usually a coronary artery, then taking a moving picture of the dye flowing through the arteries to examine the presence, location and nature of narrowings or blockages.

angioplasty: More correctly: percutaneous transluminal coronary angioplasty (PTCA). A procedure whereby a wire fitted with a deflated balloon is threaded to an area of narrowing in a coronary artery, and then inflated inside the artery to widen the artery at the point of greatest narrowing. This process is called "dilatation."

angiotensin: A substance found in the blood that causes arteries to shrink or narrow, raising blood pressure and making it more difficult for blood to flow.

angiotensin-converting enzyme inhibitors (ACE inhibitors): A type of medication that lowers blood pressure, and makes it easier for the heart to pump blood by decreasing its workload.

antiarrhythmics: Drugs used to regulate the heart rhythm. Most often these are drugs that prevent abnormally fast or irregular heartbeats from occurring.

anticoagulants: Medications that prevent the blood from clotting. Often used in patients with heart disease to prevent clots from forming inside arteries or inside heart chambers. The drug most commonly used is warfarin, which requires close monitoring by your doctor.

antidepressants: Tested medications that are of benefit to those with clinical depression. Antidepressants are always given under the supervision of a physician, who will monitor how the patient is doing. Each type of antidepressant is successful in about 70 percent of cases, so if one medication does not work, others can be tried. The problem with these medications is that they take time to work (at least a month, often more) and, especially in the first weeks, often produce side effects that may be prohibitive. However, side effects usually subside. Antidepressants need to be taken for an extended period of time. For the cardiac patient, especially soon after an event, there needs to be special attention given by and clearance obtained from the cardiologist. Monitoring is the cardinal rule of antidepressant treatment. See also *depression*.

anxiety: An unpleasant feeling we have all experienced as fear, nervousness, shakiness, worry or concern (see Chapter 10). It can also be expressed in the body as palpitations, nervous stomach and sweating, among many possibilities. It is a normal reaction to a cardiac event, but, for many, it can be ongoing. If it is within the limits of normal, often the passage of time or a recognition of it for what it is can help alleviate it. If it is ongoing, see Chapter 10. On the journey of recovery, anxiety can be complicated by the persistence of physical symptoms, creating a vicious circle. See also *fear*; *hypochondria*; *panic anxiety*.

arrhythmia: A condition in which the heart's rhythm is abnormal. Arrhythmias may cause the heart to go too fast, possibly causing palpitations, dizziness or loss of consciousness; or too slowly, resulting in weakness, lightheadedness, fatigue, dizziness or loss of consciousness.

artery: A blood vessel that carries red, oxygen-rich blood away from the heart to various body organs (including the heart, where the arteries are known as coronary arteries).

assertiveness: This term has gained more meaning in the helping professions with the finding that a firm approach in dealing with others helps to strengthen the self, for self-esteem, self-confidence and getting what you want! The term means "insisting on your rights" and is the opposite of allowing others to get their way (being *accommodating* or *submissive*) or imposing your will on others (being aggressive). (See Chapter 10.)

atherosclerosis: Hardening of the arteries. A slowly developing process in which cholesterol, scar tissue and calcium buildup occurs on the inside of arteries, gradually narrowing the size of the opening and eventually possibly leading to complete blockage.

atrial fibrillation: A non-life-threatening, somewhat rapid irregular heart rhythm that usually causes palpitations and may cause lightheadedness or shortness of breath.

autogenic relaxation: One of the relaxation techniques where there is a focus on the body, such as a muscle group (feeling hot or heavy, for example). See *relaxation techniques*.

balance or equilibrium: We use these terms to convey what must be achieved to restore health in the individual recovering from a cardiac event. This is especially so in the process of recuperation, and for recovery itself. The reason a concept such as "balance" is used is that the processes we go through and the contexts in which we live are not static, but are dynamic. Thus, when a healthy pattern has been achieved, we can say an equilibrium or balance has been restored.

beta blockers: Drugs that slow the heartbeat and can prevent heart attack recurrence. They block the action of "beta receptors," which are signal receivers on heart cells that allow adrenaline and other stress hormones to speed up the heartbeat and increase the force of its pumping.

bypass surgery: Coronary artery bypass surgery. An operation during which a bypass ("detour") is made to go around an area of blockage in a coronary artery. Bypasses are usually fashioned from veins in the legs or an artery from the inside of the chest wall. Most patients have several bypasses during a single operation, on the average two to four.

calcium channel blockers: Drugs that prevent calcium from entering cells through "calcium channels." They lower blood pressure and may weaken the pumping strength of the heart. They are very effective in decreasing angina.

cardiac arrest: A life-threatening disturbance during which the heart ceases to pump blood effectively. Usually caused by a life-threatening heart rhythm disturbance such as *ventricular fibrillation* or *ventricular tachycardia.*

cardiologist: A doctor with special training in internal medicine or diseases of various body organs, with subsequent special training in diseases of the heart. Most cardiologists train for six years after completing medical school and write several examinations before they are officially recognized as cardiologists.

cardiopulmonary resuscitation (CPR): Involves maintaining, temporarily, effective blood circulation until sophisticated care can be made available. Includes mouth-to-mouth breathing and chest compressions, which results in squeezing blood out of and letting it back into the heart. Provides some, but not normal, blood flow to the brain and heart.

cardioversion: An electrical shock delivered to the chest wall to restore normal heartbeat. Usually used for *atrial fibrillation* or *ventricular tachycardia.*

cholesterol: A fatty substance found in the blood as well as in various foods. Although necessary for life, excess cholesterol in the blood leads to a greater likelihood of *atherosclerosis* (hardening of the arteries).

clinical depression: An identifiable constellation of symptoms and signs that show that the depression has reached a point where treatment is required. There is evidence that a chemical imbalance has now occurred that needs correction; otherwise it could be many months before this type of depression lifts. The dangers of clinical depression include self-destructiveness (including suicidal tendencies) as well as ongoing unhappiness and a poor quality of life (see Joe). For depressed patients who have also had a heart attack, there is evidence that their cardiac outcome is worse than that of patients who are not clinically depressed. In sum, patients with clinical depression must receive treatment; the good news is that it is eminently treatable! See also *depression* (and Chapter 10).

clot buster: *Thrombolytic agent* that dissolves clots already formed inside blood vessels. If given early after a heart attack, it can limit the amount of damage from the heart attack and improve the chances for survival and successful recovery.

cognitive therapy: A form of psychotherapy where your thinking is changed so as to improve your feeling. Used for mild depression, it is increasingly popular, but patients should be aware that there is a work component. See also *psychotherapy*.

congestive heart failure (CHF): A condition in which the heart is too weak to pump blood effectively for the body's needs. This usually results in shortness of breath, weakness and fatigue.

coronary artery disease (CAD): Narrowings or blockages in the coronary arteries, i.e., atherosclerosis of the arteries that supply the heart with blood.

coronary artery bypass surgery: See *bypass surgery*.

Coronary Care Unit (CCU): A specialized ward in a hospital where seriously ill heart patients are kept. The unit offers close observation, close monitoring by nurses and doctors, and continuous monitoring of the *electrocardiogram (ECG)*.

coronary heart disease: Term usually used interchangeably with *coronary artery disease*.

coronary stent: A small tubular wire object inserted into a *coronary artery* at the time of *angioplasty* to keep the previously narrowed artery open and to hold it open for the long term. Usually done in conjunction with *PTCA*.

deep breathing: The "mother" of relaxation techniques, involving deep, slow, controlled breathing. It is similar to the breathing component of yoga. An abdominal component adds to its power. See also *relaxation techniques*.

defibrillation: An electrical shock, usually delivered to the chest wall, using paddles to restore heartbeat to normal in case of life-threatening rapid heart rhythms (*ventricular fibrillation*).

denial: Specifically in this book, the shutting out of concerns about heart disease and simply "getting on with it." The crucial point is *whether you are following your treatment program*! As long as you are, your denial can be considered "adaptive," and is usually an acceptable part of making a recovery, although you *will* benefit from being actively aware of your condition. If you are not following treatment recommendations, your denial is "maladaptive," which is actively discouraged.

depression: General term referring to a variety of feelings or conditions related to low mood. Includes sadness, low mood, clinical depression and persistent low mood (see individual entries).

diabetes: A condition in which there is too much sugar in the bloodstream; the condition is associated with a higher risk of coronary heart disease. Usually treated with insulin or blood sugar–lowering drugs.

disorientation: Specifically in this book, a state of mild *emotional* confusion or disorientation (people don't "feel themselves") often experienced during the aftermath phase. This is not to be confused(!) with real confusion or disorientation; it merely describes an "in-between state" that usually resolves itself within a few days, although for some it can linger (see Chapter 4).

echocardiogram: An ultrasound or "radar" image of the heart. A simple painless procedure during which the heart image is stored on videotape for later review. Accurate pictures are obtained that allow detailed examination of the heart's interior.

electrocardiogram (ECG): A test of the electrical activity of the heart, recorded from electrodes (sticky buttons) placed on the limbs and chest. An electrocardiogram is very useful in searching for prior heart damage, lack of blood supply to the heart, and heart rhythm disturbances.

empowerment: Strength that emerges once you have mastery over what you do. In the journey of recovery, this classically occurs in the early part of rehabilitation, when patients realize that they *can do* things; this is invariably associated with structured activity that is the hallmark of the rehabilitation programs.

exercise: Physical activity that improves the ability of the heart and the body to perform work. *Isotonic exercise* involves moving the body through space, such as walking, jogging, bicycling and swimming. *Isometric exercise* involves trying to overcome a resistance, such as weight lifting, push-ups and other strengthening exercises. Both types are beneficial in patients with heart disease.

exercise test: A test during which patients do exercise with a specific difficulty, at a given pace under close medical supervision. An *electrocardiogram* is always recorded continuously during this test. The exercise may involve walking or jogging on a treadmill, or riding a bicycle; the difficulty of the exercise is increased progressively until the heart rate reaches a predefined maximum, or until the patient can no longer carry on. This test is used to look for *myocardial ischemia* or *arrhythmias*, and to test fitness level.

event: Specifically in this book, what has occurred to signify *coronary artery disease*. This would include a *heart attack*, *bypass surgery*, *angioplasty* or even a symptom such as *angina,* which heralds the diagnosis of CAD. It is the first of the series of phases in the journey of recovery. See also *phases*.

fear: An unpleasant feeling, universally experienced, when there is a threat present or perceived. It is often distinguished from anxiety by being directly related to a specific feared object (such as a charging lion), but the term is commonly used in a looser way, as generalized fear, in which case it can safely be called anxiety. Fear is a normal response while experiencing or having experienced a cardiac event, and especially in respect of concern about something threatening happening in the future (such as a *heart attack*). See also *anxiety*.

hardening of the arteries: See *atherosclerosis*.

heart attack: A specific event during which portions of the heart muscle are deprived of blood for sufficiently long that the muscle cells die. Results in permanent heart damage, of varying severity. Almost always caused by temporary or permanent complete blockage of a coronary artery.

Holter monitoring: Continuous monitoring of an *electrocardiogram* (*ECG*), usually for twenty-four or more hours, by recording all of the ECG (heartbeats) onto a cassette recorder worn over the shoulder or on a belt, for later playback into a computer and detailed analysis. Useful in assessing patients with *myocardial ischemia* or *arrhythmias*.

hostility: One of the manifestations of anger. It has a particularly "nasty" quality, implying that the anger is specifically directed at someone or some entity. Hostility is outwardly directed, and so is observed by others and often invites a response. This response, naturally, can be hostile as well, giving rise to "hostilities." The book title *Anger Kills* (by Redford Williams and Virginia Williams) thus has a double meaning, as hostility can harm others as well as the cardiac patient, for whom it is a risk factor for CAD. See also *anger*.

hypervigilance: Specifically in this book, an exaggeration of the normal protective response of the family, usually the spouse, when the patient returns home from the hospital after *heart attack* or *cardiac arrest*. There is scrutiny as the loved one is fearful that "something will happen" to the patient. Hypervigilance usually subsides fairly rapidly; otherwise it can cause problems for the patient and significant others (see Chapter 4).

hypochondria: The tendency for concern or fear that one will develop a serious disease. We use this term for those patients during the emotional reaction of recuperation after a cardiac event who, in spite of reassurances from their physicians, are inordinately concerned about a worsening of their condition, to the extent that it dominates their lives. See also *anxiety*.

imaging: One of the *relaxation techniques*. It involves imagining a scene that is relaxing to you. It is helpful initially for the relaxation therapist to describe a scene, so as to assist you to learn "how to do it." Ultimately, we prefer that you create your own scene to provide a focus for the relaxation technique. See also *stress management*; *visualization*.

Intensive Care Unit (ICU): Similar to a *Coronary Care Unit*, but may have critically ill patients with non-heart-related problems. Following *bypass*, most patients stay in a cardiovascular intensive care unit for one to several days as part of the normal recovery from surgery.

ischemia: See *myocardial ischemia*.

isometric exercise. See *exercise*.

isotonic exercise. See *exercise*.

low mood: A loose term used to describe any mood that is low or negative; in this context, we are referring especially to a period during recuperation when the mind reacts to the feeling of incapacity; this coincides with early healing of the body, when it is natural for patients to feel fatigued or generally "not themselves." The feeling of not being capable is associated with low mood. The converse is true as well. When patients feel that they are capable, the mood goes up again. This is typically seen during the rehabilitation phase. See also *depression*.

maintenance: Specifically in this book, what is required *after* the journey of recovery. It is important for the patient to maintain heart-healthy habits in order to prevent slippage and possible recurrence. This challenge is usually underestimated (see Chapter 7).

meditation: One of the main relaxation techniques. It can be the most difficult to learn, but is often the most rewarding once mastered. The focus here is the "mantra" derived from transcendental meditation, which is repetitive and has no specific meaning. Defocusing or shutting intrusive thoughts out can be difficult, but once it is achieved, the relaxation response occurs. Meditation is often found to be difficult for those with active minds (see Mary), but again, if obstacles are overcome, it can be very effective. See also *relaxation techniques*.

myocardial infarction: See *heart attack*.

myocardial ischemia: A condition in which there is insufficient blood and oxygen supply to the heart muscle. It may, but does not have to, be associated with *angina*. During myocardial ischemia, the *electrocardiogram* (*ECG*) is usually abnormal.

nitroglycerin: A drug which dilates blood vessels and, when taken under the tongue (sublingually) or sprayed to the back of the throat, results in prompt relief of angina.

nuclear angiogram (thallium or Cardiolite® scan): A test during which a small amount of radioactive substance is injected into an arm vein and the patient is subjected to exercise or a drug that stresses the heart. Pictures or images are then taken of the heart and indicate if parts of the heart muscle get insufficient blood supply or are scarred.

obesity: A condition characterized by being overweight and carrying excess body fat. Obesity is known to contribute to high blood pressure, diabetes, and the likelihood of heart attack and death.

occupational therapist: A person with a university degree who is qualified to assist people recover from physical or emotional conditions through activity and programs. Occupational therapists can be invaluable in helping cardiac patients by teaching *stress management*.

panic anxiety or panic disorder: Panic is a special form of anxiety; it is intense, and can be felt directly or, commonly, expressed through bodily sensations such as palpitations, chest pain and dizziness. It is often associated with alarming thoughts such as that one is "going to die," "lose control" or "have a heart attack." Repeated panic attacks or panic disorder can occur in *CAD* patients and can be confusing to diagnose. Anyone with initial or persistent panic symptoms must see his or her physician. See also *anxiety*.

pericarditis: A condition in which the lining of the heart is inflamed. Often accompanies a heart attack or can occur after *bypass surgery*. May cause shortness of breath, chest discomfort or fever.

persistent low mood: A low mood or depression, not severe enough to be a clinical depression, that persists over time. There is accumulating evidence to show that patients with persistent low mood do worse than others after heart attack. Not only do they benefit from relief from this condition, but they can expect a better cardiac outcome. See also *depression*.

phases: The concept of distinct periods of time used in this book to assist patients to recover after a cardiac event. We have emphasized that the phases do overlap, especially recuperation and rehabilitation, but that thinking about them separately does help you to understand and better deal with what you are going through. See also *aftermath*; *event*; *recovery*; *recuperation*; *rehabilitation*.

platelets: Tiny blood elements that can stick or "clump" together, blocking arteries on their own, or leading to formation of clots, which can block an artery.

progressive muscular relaxation: One of the relaxation techniques; it involves tensing and relaxing muscle groups up and down the body. It is often useful to initiate a sequence of relaxation techniques and is also good "in the field," especially for those who are tense. See *relaxation techniques*.

psychiatrist: A physician who has qualified as a specialist to deal with emotional difficulties or mental illness generally. A psychiatrist can prescribe medications.

psychologist: A qualified person with a doctoral degree, specializing in emotional difficulties. A cardiac psychologist will have special expertise with cardiac patients; for example, in cognitive therapy.

psychotherapy: Treatment of difficulties by talking or other psychological methods. See also *cognitive therapy*; *supportive therapy*.

PTCA. See *angioplasty*.

reactive: More liable to respond to what goes on in the environment. The reactive person is invariably a sensitive person. For sensitive cardiac patients and their families, it is important to be aware of these tendencies, so as to be able to deal with stress, which can be more difficult for such people than for those who are less sensitive. The learning of stress-management skills is recommended for the sensitive and reactive person. (See also *sensitivity* and Chapter 10.)

reconstruction: Reconstruction, or rebuilding, is what is going on from an emotional point of view during the rehabilitation phase. See also *rehabilitation*.

recovery: The final phase in the journey of recovery, implying a return to health (see Chapter 7). We distinguish here between recovery from the cardiac event, from the experience itself and, what is more controversial, from *coronary artery disease* itself.

recuperation: The third phase in the journey of recovery. In this relatively long phase (lasting at least months), the body heals, but at the same time the mind initially reacts. Recuperation concludes with the establishment of balance in the body and mind, and other aspects of the person's life, including the family system. See also *phases*.

rehabilitation: The fourth phase in the journey of recovery. A long (lasting at least months) phase characterized by a focus on structured activity epitomized by the programs, particularly those with an exercise base, which have greatly enhanced the quality of life in *CAD* patients. See also *phases*.

relaxation response: This was originally described by Herbert Benson as the response that occurred to a relaxation technique characterized by using a focused activity and allowing, at the same time, other thoughts to be shut out of the mind. The response is one that is both mental and physical—that of relaxation. See also *relaxation techniques*.

relaxation techniques: Techniques that have been designed to elicit the relaxation response in those who are anxious. A sequence is chosen, and practiced on a regular basis. See also *autogenic relaxation*; *deep breathing*; *imaging*; *visualization*; *meditation*; *progressive muscular relaxation*; *relaxation response*.

risk-factor modification: Attempts to reduce the impact of factors such as high cholesterol, smoking, sedentary living, diabetes and high blood pressure, which have been found to affect the course of *coronary heart disease*.

sadness: The normal response to loss. In the early part of recovering from a cardiac event, it is normal to experience sadness due to perceived losses. While some losses, such as now being a "heart patient," will remain, many of the losses turn out to be perceived (and not real). See also *depression*; *low mood* (and Chapter 5).

sensitivity: A tendency seen in those persons who do not ignore the incoming stimuli of the environment and so are more affected by what happens. Dealing with stress is a challenge for sensitive patients, especially as their sensitivity is associated with being reactive. Patients and their families who are sensitive and reactive should be aware of these tendencies, and develop stress-management skills to deal not only with what will occur on the journey of recovery, but with what awaits them on the other journeys of their lives. See also *reactive* (and Chapter 10).

social support: Almost all of us need emotional support, but for the cardiac patient, social support has been found to improve *CAD* outcome. The source of social support that has the most benefit has not been identified, but we feel that all types of support are welcome! A mainstay of our lives is the relationship with a confidante, often a spouse. But any supportive social network, as well as the social activities, has also been found to have benefit for the cardiac patient. Emotional support can also be obtained through either individual or group therapy (see Chapter 10).

social worker: A person trained to deal with problems and situations of an interpersonal nature. For the cardiac patient, the social worker is often invaluable in the inpatient setting, for those with social and family problems. For outpatients, social workers can assist with family problems, ongoing social support and therapy.

somatic: A bodily response. For example, anxiety can have its somatic form as muscle tension, nervous stomach, palpitations and many other manifestations. Depression can be expressed in a somatic form as, say, fatigue. It has been observed that those who have difficulty facing up to their emotional problems are more likely to have somatic complaints.

stress: A very loose term referring to excessive pressure or demand. It is this implication of being excessive that makes stress difficult to define, as what is too much for some can be just right, or even easily manageable, for others. Other terms associated with stress are also used in a rather loose way. The *stressor* is that which causes or initiates the stress. *Distress* is the unpleasant feeling we get when we are under stress. It is important for patient and family to be able to deal with the expected and unexpected stressors on the journey of recovery; if you find it difficult to manage, you should be looking at and learning stress-management techniques. See *stress management* (and Chapter 10).

stress management: Broadly, attempts to deal with stress. The specific approaches have been refined as stress-management techniques. After a cardiac event, much of what patients and their families go through emotionally is a normal response to the event; if, however, the experience is severe or prolonged, you will require management for it. We have explained when to seek professional advice, for example, in the case of clinical depression. Otherwise, you may well benefit from learning stress-management techniques. For the cardiac patient, there is an extra incentive as certain tendencies have been held to affect the course of CAD. The usual techniques that apply to cardiac patients are relaxation techniques and anger and time management. See also *anger management*; *relaxation techniques*; *time management* (and Chapter 10).

submissive: The tendency to yield to others; allowing others to get their way. Submissive is similar to being *accommodating*, but to an extreme. The problem with being submissive for cardiac patients is that they are more likely to take on an excessive burden and so be stressed, unlike more *assertive* people. Many patients and spouses are overloaded at home and at work. They can benefit from being assertive; but being submissive is often a long-standing, even lifelong, tendency and naturally this can be difficult to change. Assertiveness training can be of great benefit to the accommodating or submissive person. See also *accommodating*; *assertiveness* (and Chapter 10).

thrombolytic agent: See *clot buster*.

time management: Specifically in this book, techniques developed for the cardiac patient based on the assumption that the cardiac patient can be a time-pressured individual. Such people are more at risk for stress-related problems. Time-pressured individuals are easily put in an overload situation when "one more thing" is added to their busy schedules, especially if this thing is a cardiac event! Time-management techniques can be helpful for such people. See also *stress management* (and Chapter 10).

tranquilizers: A group of medications used to calm down patients, and often given in the inpatient setting. The medications do work, and are not usually toxic to the heart at all. However, this is a problem with their continued use, which can lead to dependence, and withdrawal on discontinuation. This is particularly true of the short-acting variety (those that only last a few hours in the body). Tranquilizers must be obtained from a physician, and, as is true of all medications, monitoring is the key.

unstable angina: *Angina* that occurs at rest, or lasts for prolonged periods (e.g., longer than thirty minutes) and does not get better after *nitroglycerin.* Almost always leads to hospitalization. Can be considered a "threatened heart attack."

ventricular fibrillation: A life-threatening, abnormal, very rapid heart rhythm during which the heart "quivers" and does not pump blood effectively. Causes death within minutes unless CPR is administered and the patient is *defibrillated.*

ventricular tachycardia: A rapid, usually regular and dangerous heart rhythm. May cause loss of consciousness and require urgent electrical shock (*cardioversion*) to restore the normal heartbeat.

visualization: The creation in your mind of an image or a situation. For the cardiac patient, visualization involves creating a series of linked images in the mind to help empower you to overcome CAD. We do not emphasize visualization, but prefer to incorporate the imaging component as a stress-management technique for cardiac patients. See also *imaging*; *relaxation techniques.*

Index

Accommodating person, 235
ACE inhibitors, 60, 169–72
Acetylsalicylic acid (ASA), 59, 172, 186, 187, 253
Active participation in treatment, 261
Activities:
  after hospital discharge, 42
  readiness for, 263–64
  in recuperation period, 55, 61–63
Acute congestive heart failure, 159
Adaptive denial, 92–93, 242, 277
Adrenaline, 59, 60, 173
Aftermath, 12–13, 38–51
  Anna, 270–71
  changes in life, 38–39
  discharge from hospital, 40–42, 50–51
  disorientation, 43–45, 49
  family concerns, 45–47, 48–49
  Kevin, 284–85
  resumption of activities, 42
  Tony, 266–67
Aggression, 71, 227–29, 235, 236
Alcohol, 194
Anger:
  assertiveness training, 228, 236, 273
  management of, 108, 228–29, 272, 273
  in recuperation, 70–72, 135, 137, 272, 287
  risk factor for heart attack, 70, 217, 218, 226–27
Anger Kills, 109, 228, 236, 290
Angina:
  cause of, 25, 150
  defined, 25, 294
  stable, 25
  unstable, 26
Angina pectoris, 58
Angiogram, 47, 55–56, 78, 161
Angiography. *see* Coronary angiography
Angioplasty. *see* Percutaneous transluminal coronary angioplasty (PTCA)
Angiotensin, 60, 170
Anna:
  aftermath, 270–71
  forum, 32–37
  recovery, 273–74
  recuperation, 271–72
  rehabilitation, 273
Antiarrhythmic drugs, 61
Anticoagulants. *see* Blood thinners
Antidepressants, 69–70, 281, 282
Anxiety:
  after discharge from hospital, 40, 41, 135
  effects, 257, 271–72
  interaction with physical symptoms, 65, 146, 254–55

in recuperation, 65, 206–10
two forms, 207–8
worry about another cardiac event or dying, 218
Arrhythmias, 151, 153–58
after a heart attack, 58–59
less serious, 153–54
medications against, 61, 116–17
serious forms, 154–55
treatment of serious forms, 155–56
Arteries:
cerebral (brain), 151–52
coronary (to heart), 25, 150, 163
formation of clots in. *see* Blood clots
Aspirin, 59, 161, 172
Assertiveness, 116, 119–20, 223, 234–36, 282–83
training, 228, 235, 236, 273
Atherosclerosis:
contributing factors, 97, 137
and high blood pressure, 200
process, 25, 149, 150
slow development, 104, 128
Atria, 153
Atrial fibrillation, 116, 117, 151, 157
controlling by medications, 177–78
"Attachment," 220
Attitude:
in aftermath, 39, 51
effect on heart, 18
optimism in recuperation, 75–76
positive attitude important to recovery, 128, 129, 133, 277
in rehabilitation, 104, 109–10
Autogenic relaxation, 225
Awareness, forum, 16–20
• • •
Baker, Dr Brian, introduced, 7
Balance, 13–14, 53, 54, 124, 229, 258–59
keeping a balance, 131–34
"road smoothing" in recuperation, 73–77
Balloon angioplasty. *see* Percutaneous transluminal coronary angioplasty (PTCA)
Belief system, 218
Benson, Herbert, 107–8, 224
Beta blockers, 59, 60, 161, 172–74
Blockage. *see* Occlusion of artery
Blood clots, 150, 152
in arteries to the brain, 151–52
formation in coronary arteries, 25, 150
medications and, 26, 157, 160–61, 170, 174–76
in other body organs, 152
prevention by aspirin, 59
Blood pressure, lowering after a heart attack, 60
Blood thinners, 157, 174–76
Bypass surgery, 26, 56, 167–68, 253
• • •
Caffeine, 194–95
Calcium antagonists, 176
Calcium channel blockers, 61
Cardiac arrest, 51, 155, 159
Cardiac catheterization, 162–64
Cardiologists, 182–83
Cardiopulmonary resuscitation (CPR), 155–56, 159
Cardioversion, 154
Cardioverter defibrillator, implanted, 157

Cholesterol:
- damage to arteries, 190
- and exercise, 197
- and family history, 199
- lowering by medications, 60–61, 79, 103, 176–77, 189–90
- lowering through diet, 61, 102–3
- risk factor, 188–90

Clinical depression, 68–70, 85–86, 249, 262, 281–82
- and CAD, 212–13
- evaluation and treatment, 114, 117, 213–14
- meaning, 212

Clot busters, 26, 160–61, 176
- clinical trials of, 185
- development, 184–85

Clots. *see* Blood clots
Cognitive therapy, 69, 70, 209, 213, 214, 282
Collaterals, 57
Competitiveness, 227
Compliance with treatment, 77, 106–7, 133, 250
- effect of depression, 115
- slippage, 113, 269

Confidantes, 231, 232
Congestive heart failure, 58, 90–91, 153
Connotation, 257
Controlled clinical trial, 185–88
Coronary angiography, 27, 162, 163, 253
Coronary arteries, 25, 150, 163
Coronary artery disease (CAD)
- defined, 297
- factors causing. *see* Risk factors
- hope for reversal, 124
- hospitalization and treatment, 160–62

Coronary bypass surgery, 26, 56, 167–68, 253
Coronary care units (CCUs), 26, 31, 161
Coronary stents, 57, 169
Counseling for emotional problems, 242–45

• • •

Damasio, Dr Antonio, 90, 249, 292
Dance of Anger, 30, 291
Deep breathing, 225
Defibrillation, 47, 154, 156, 159
Defocusing, 224
Delayed response, 63
Demands and losses, 220
Denial. *see* Adaptive denial; Maladaptive denial
Denotation, 256–57
Depression, 146, 210–15, 262, 278–79, 281–82
- clinical. *see* Clinical depression
- effect on compliance, 115
- mild (low mood), 67–68, 70, 81
- persistent low mood, 67, 214–15

Descartes' Error, 90, 249, 292
Diabetes, risk factor, 191, 200
Diet:
- changing philosophy toward eating, 103
- lowering cholesterol through, 61, 102–103
- risk factor, 191–95
- sticking to, 118–19

Dietitians, 183
Digoxin, 177–78
Disability payments, 96

Discharge from hospital, 40–42, 50–51
Discordance, 43–45
Disorientation, 43–45, 49
Distress, 220–21
Diuretics ("water pills"), 153, 178
Dizziness:
  after time of discharge, 41–42
  in recuperation period, 58, 59
Doctors:
  cardiologists, 182–83
  family doctors, 181–82, 243, 273, 281
  following doctor's orders. *see* Compliance with treatment
  other specialists, 183–84, 242–45
Dorian, Dr Paul, introduced, 7–8

• • •

Echocardiogram, 27, 161, 164
Ejection fraction, 134
Electrical shock to restore heartbeat, 154, 156, 159
Electrocardiogram (ECG), 160, 164–65
  in CCUs, 31
Electrophysiologic study, 165
Embolus, 152
Emergency, 158–59
Emotions:
  during heart attack, 23–24, 28–31, 37
  expressing, 82–83
  professional counseling, 107, 112–13, 132, 242–45
  reactions during recuperation, 13, 63–72
  see also Adaptive denial; Anger; Anxiety; Attitude; Depression; Fear; Loss; Low mood; Motivation; Panic; Sadness; Stress; Stress management
Empowerment:
  four steps, 94
  through structured activity, 94–95
Equanimity:
  ten steps to, 131–34
  see also Balance
Erikson, Dr Erik, 218
Estrogen, 203, 204–5
Event, 12, 21–37
  coping with (forum), 32–37
  Kevin, 283–84
  Tony, 265–66
Exercise:
  benefits, 197, 199
  commitment, 198–99
  and effect of heart damage, 58
  and heart failure, 90–91
  heart rate and, 60, 174
  isometric, 101–2, 198
  isotonic, 100–1, 198
  lowering blood pressure by, 171, 197
  in rehabilitation, 87, 100–2, 119, 195
  setting goals, 199
  and social support, 196
  as stress management, 107
Exercise physiologists, 183
Exercise testing, 27, 42, 55, 78, 162, 165, 263
Expressing emotions, 82–83
Extended shock phase, 30

• • •

Family, 37, 39, 43
  belonging to a team, 132

see also Significant others; Spouse
Family concerns, 45–47, 48–49
in the aftermath, 45–47
in recuperation, 72–73, 78–84
in rehabilitation, 98–100, 110–11
Family counseling, 245, 276
Family doctor, 181–82, 243, 273, 281
Family history, risk factor, 78, 81–82, 97, 199–200
Fatigue:
and depression, 256, 262
emotions and, 76–77, 89, 256
Fear:
in aftermath, 40
in recuperation, 64–65, 286
see also Anxiety
Fibrates, 177
Fish in diet, 193
Focusing the mind for relaxation, 108
techniques, 224–25
Folic acid, 97
Forum:
awareness, 16–20
dealing with the event, 32–37
finding the path of healing, 78–84
getting into gear, 113–20
looking back and looking forward, 134–40
lost and found, 47–51
Friendships, 110, 119, 232
• • •
Habits:
changing, 75–76, 88, 98, 104, 127, 129–30, 133, 134, 269
heart-healthy habits, 14–15, 19, 104, 130
unhealthy habits, 18, 128
Hardening of the arteries. *see* Atherosclerosis
Healing. *see* Recuperation
Heart attack:
activities after. *see* Activities
aftermath. *see* Aftermath
causes, 24–26, 150
changes in life following, 38–39, 53, 83–84
damage from, 58, 150, 152–53
emotional experience, 23–24, 27–31, 37, 63
event. *see* Event
importance of prompt treatment, 26
indication on ECG, 160
phases from event through recovery, 4–5, 11, 12–15
physical experience, 21, 23
problems following, 58
recovery. *see* Recovery
recuperation. *see* Recuperation
recurring attacks, 21–22, 29–30, 33–37
reducing severity by “clot busters,” 160–61
rehabilitation. *see* Rehabilitation
response, 6, 28–31, 37
Heart disease, defined, 149
Heart failure, 151, 153
and exercise, 90–91
Heart rate:
and beta blockers, 173–74
and exercise, 60, 174
increased by anger or emotional upset, 60
Heartmates, 100, 290
Heparin, 161, 174–75

High blood pressure:
- and atherosclerosis, 200
- medications, 201
- risk factors, 200–201

High-density lipoproteins (HDLs), 189
Holter monitoring, 116, 165–66
Homocysteine, 97
Hospitals:
- admission to, 26, 160–62
- CCUs in. *see* Coronary care units (CCUs)
- discharge from, 40, 41, 50–51
- stay in, 31–32, 39–40, 41
- survival rate in, 27

Humor and laughter, 111–12
Hunter, John, 217
Hypertension. *see* High blood pressure
Hypervigilance, 13, 46, 48–49, 73, 136, 285
Hypochondria, 207, 208, 209

• • •

Imaging, 225
Impotence, 62–63
Infarction. *see* Heart attack
Insulin, 191
International normalized ratio (INR), 175
Intimacy, 62
- *see also* Sexual activity

Ischemia. *see* Myocardial ischemia
Isometric exercise, 101–2, 198
Isotonic exercise, 100–1, 198

• • •

Joe, 28, 256, 281–83
- clinical depression, 68–70, 85–86, 114
- recovery, 282–83
- rehabilitation, 85–86, 113–20

• • •

Kevin, 233, 257
- aftermath, 284–85
- event, 283–84
- recovery, 121–23, 134–40
- recuperation, 285–87
- rehabilitation, 287–88

Kidneys, 170

• • •

Left ventricular function, 58
Lerner, Harriet, 30
Lipoproteins, 189
Liver, and cholesterol, 189, 192
Longevity, effects of exercise, 197
Loss, 65–67, 275
Low blood pressure, and ACE inhibitors, 169–72
Low mood, 67–68, 70, 81, 262, 268, 278
- persistent low mood, 214–15

Low-density lipoproteins (LDLs), 177, 189

• • •

Maintenance, 127–30, 132–33
Maladaptive denial, 93, 96, 115
Mary, 52–53, 254, 278–81
- recovery, 280–81
- recuperation, 78–84, 278–79
- rehabilitation, 279

Medical research, 184–88
Medical treatment, 160–69
- surgical procedures, 167–69
- tests, 156, 160, 161, 162–67

Medications:
- antidepressants, 69–70
- for arrhythmia, 116–17

clinical depression, 213–14
compliance (taking as prescribed), 77, 106–107, 113, 133, 180–81, 250, 253, 269
control, not cure, 125
for depression, 117
general advice about, 179–81
high blood pressure, 103, 201
recuperation, 57, 59–61, 69–70
routines for taking, 42, 181
specific medications, 169–79
to lower cholesterol, 103
Meditation, 225, 230
Mediterranean diet, 193
Mistrustfulness, 270, 272
Monitoring, 125
Motivation, 20, 129, 267, 269
MUGA scan, 166
Myocardial enzymes, 161
Myocardial infarction. *see* Heart attack
Myocardial ischemia, 151, 160, 161
defined, 300–301
diagnosed by exercise tests, 165
symptoms, 25
• • •
Natural bypasses (collaterals), 57
Nitrates, 161, 179
Nitroglycerin, 37, 61, 178–79
Noncompliance, 113, 115, 269
Normal heartbeat, 157–58
Nuclear imaging, 166–67
Nurses, 184
• • •
Obesity, risk factors, 201–2
Occlusion of artery, 25
reducing the risk following PTCA, 57
Optimism. *see* Positive attitude
Osteoporosis, 205
• • •
Pacemaker:
artificial, 158
natural, 157–58
Pacing of activities, 230, 279
Panic, 245
panic disorder, 208, 209
Patience, 133
Perception of a symptom, 256–57
Percutaneous transluminal coronary angioplasty (PTCA), 26, 33, 56–57, 79, 168–69, 253
defined, 3, 294
Pericarditis, 41
Persistent low mood, 67, 214–15
Pessimists, 220
see also Positive attitude; Stress management
Platelets:
and clotting, 161, 170
prevention of clumping by aspirin, 59
see also Blood clots
"Plumbing" problems following a heart attack, 58
Positive attitude, 51, 104, 109–10, 128, 129, 133, 277
Post-traumatic response, 29, 30–31
Premature ventricular contractions (extra beats), 58
Professional advice for emotional problems, 107, 112–13, 132, 242–45
Professional rescue, 156
Progressive muscular relaxation, 225

Protectiveness, 43, 46–47, 48–49, 136, 270
Psychiatric emergency, 245
Psychiatrists, 183–84
Psychological well-being, measuring, 247, 248
Psychologists, 183
Psychotherapy, 108–9, 209, 244, 245, 282
Pulmonary embolus, 152
"Pushiness," 227–29, 235

• • •

Reactivity, 233–34, 257, 285–87
Realism, 134
Reconstruction, emotional, 87, 91–92
Recovery, 14–15, 121–41
  Anna, 273–74
  family, 130
  forum on, 134–40
  Joe, 282–83
  Kevin, 121–23, 134–40
  maintenance, 127–30, 132–33
  Mary, 280–81
  realistic, 125–26
  Rose, 276–77
  ten steps to equanimity, 131–34
  Tony, 269–70
Recuperation, 13–14, 254, 258
  activities, 61–63
  Anna, 271–72
  bodily healing, 54–55
  changing undesirable habits, 75–76
  depression. *see* Depression
  emotional healing, 63–72
  family matters, 72–73, 78–84
  "fork in the road," 75
  further medical procedures, 56–57
  Kevin, 285–87
  Mary, 278–79
  meaning, 252–53
  medications, 57, 59–61, 69–70, 77
  problems, 58–59
  restoring a balance, 73–77
  Rose, 275
  social activities, 77
  Tony, 267–68
Recurrences of heart problems, 21–22, 33–37
Rehabilitation, 14, 253, 258
  adaptive denial, 92–93
  Anna, 273
  bodily sensations during, 89–90
  exercise, 100–2
  family concerns, 98–100, 110–11
  from reaction to reconstruction, 91–92
  increasing understanding, 103–4
  individual needs, 98
  Joe, 85–86
  Kevin, 287–88
  Mary, 279
  meanings, 86–87
  medications, 103, 106–7, 113
  modifying behavior to minimize risk, 88, 97–98, 102–3
  perspective on, 88–89
  readiness for, 260–64
  Rose, 275–76
  slippage, 112–13
  stress management, 105–12
  structured activities, 86, 87–88, 94–96
  Tony, 268–69
Relaxation:
  "relaxation response," 107–8

techniques, 108, 209, 210, 223–26, 230, 244
see also Stress management
Religion, 110, 111
Reopening of the coronary arteries, 124
Restenosis, 57
Risk factors, 188–203
cholesterol. *see* Cholesterol
diabetes, 191, 200
diet, 191–95
examples, 97
family history, 78, 81–82, 97, 199–200
high blood pressure (hypertension), 200–1
modifying, 75–76, 88, 97–98, 102–3, 128
obesity, 201–2
smoking. *see* Smoking
Rose, 38–39, 47–51, 231–32, 275–77
recovery, 276–77
recuperation, 275
rehabilitation, 275–76

• • •

Sadness, 66–67, 275, 278
Salt, and diuretics, 178
Saturated fats, 189
Scarring following a heart attack, 58, 150, 152–53
Scientific approach, 248
Self-control, 230, 234
Sensitivity, 233–34, 257
Sexual activity, 263, 268
after hospital discharge, 42
impotence, 62–63
and length of life, 62
in recuperation period, 61, 62–63
Shock response, 28–31, 31–32, 37
extended shock phase, 30
Sick role, 92, 261
Significant others
in aftermath, 39
anxiety, 210
during event, 266, 284
effects on, 36, 274
support for, 99, 100
see also Spouse
Sinoatrial node, 157–58
Slippage, 112–13, 126, 127–28, 130, 269
Slow heartbeats, 157–58
Smoking:
risk factor, 202
stopping, 76, 202–3, 267
Social activities:
in aftermath, 42
in recuperation, 77
Social support, 110–11, 119, 219, 230–32
and exercise, 196
Somatic amplification, 255
Spirituality and health, 110, 111, 218
Spouse:
in aftermath, 45–47, 270–71, 285
during an event, 32, 35–36, 266, 284
effects of heart attack on, 35–36, 136, 274
importance in recovery, 130, 269
protectiveness, 46–47, 48–49
in recuperation, 72–73, 268, 272
support for, 99, 100
support from, in rehabilitation, 111, 120
see also Significant others

Stable angina, 25
Statins, 177, 189–90
Stenting, 57, 169
Stress, 173, 239–40
  avoiding overload, 221–23
  avoiding overreactions, 105–6
  and CAD, 88, 146, 216–19
  compliance with treatment, 106–7
  definition, 216, 304
  and high blood pressure, 200
  ongoing demands, 217
  "pacing," 106
  personal view of stress and heart disease, 237–41
  reaction, 216–17
Stress hormones, 59–60
Stress management, 99, 219–36, 240
  relaxation techniques for anxiety, 223–26, 230
  seven areas of vulnerability, 221–36
  "Ten Commandments" of, 105–12
Stroke, 151, 152
Structured activities, 86, 87–88, 94–96
Submissiveness, 235
Suicide, 245
Support group, 276
Surgical procedures, 167–69
Symptoms, 271
  awareness in recovery, 132
  discomfort after discharge, 43, 44
  during rehabilitation, 89–90
  need for further treatment, 78–79
  reasons for seeking medical help, 160
Syndrome X, 191

• • •

Tachycardia. *see* Ventricular tachycardia
Talking treatments for depression. *see* Cognitive therapy
Tests, 156, 160, 161, 162–67, 258
  prior to discharge, 27
Thrombolytic agents. *see* Clot busters
Thrombosis, 151
Time management, 229–30
Time pressure, 109, 230
Tissue damage. *see* Scarring following a heart attack
Tony:
  aftermath, 266–67
  event, 265–66
  forum, 16–20
  maladaptive denial, 93
  recovery, 269–70
  recuperation, 267–68
  rehabilitation, 268–69
Tranquilizer, 209
Transient ischemic attacks (TIAs), 152
Triglycerides, 191
Type A personality, 217–18, 226–27

• • •

Ultrasound tests, 27, 164
Unstable angina, 26, 162
  defined, 3, 305
  testing for, 55–56

• • •

Valvular regurgitation, 163
Veins, 152
Ventricles, 153
Ventricular arrhythmias, 153–54
Ventricular fibrillation, 155, 156, 158–59

Ventricular tachycardia, 58, 151, 154–55, 159
Vitamin E, 193
Vocational rehabilitation, 96
• • •
Walking, 197
Warfarin, 157, 175
Weakness by time of discharge, 41
Weight loss, 192, 202
Williams, Redford, 218, 290
Williams, Virginia, 218, 290
Women
heart disease, 203–5
signs of heart disease, 37
Work, 264
return to, 87–88, 95–96
• • •
X-ray imaging, 27